S0-BPY-947

DAC Guidelines and Reference Series

Poverty and Health

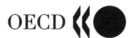
OECD

ORGANISATION FOR ECONOMIC CO-OPERATION AND DEVELOPMENT
WORLD HEALTH ORGANIZATION

RA418.5
P6
P68
2003

ORGANISATION FOR ECONOMIC CO-OPERATION AND DEVELOPMENT

Pursuant to Article 1 of the Convention signed in Paris on 14th December 1960, and which came into force on 30th September 1961, the Organisation for Economic Co-operation and Development (OECD) shall promote policies designed:

- to achieve the highest sustainable economic growth and employment and a rising standard of living in member countries, while maintaining financial stability, and thus to contribute to the development of the world economy;
- to contribute to sound economic expansion in member as well as non-member countries in the process of economic development; and
- to contribute to the expansion of world trade on a multilateral, non-discriminatory basis in accordance with international obligations.

The original member countries of the OECD are Austria, Belgium, Canada, Denmark, France, Germany, Greece, Iceland, Ireland, Italy, Luxembourg, the Netherlands, Norway, Portugal, Spain, Sweden, Switzerland, Turkey, the United Kingdom and the United States. The following countries became members subsequently through accession at the dates indicated hereafter: Japan (28th April 1964), Finland (28th January 1969), Australia (7th June 1971), New Zealand (29th May 1973), Mexico (18th May 1994), the Czech Republic (21st December 1995), Hungary (7th May 1996), Poland (22nd November 1996), Korea (12th December 1996) and the Slovak Republic (14th December 2000). The Commission of the European Communities takes part in the work of the OECD (Article 13 of the OECD Convention).

In order to achieve its aims the OECD has set up a number of specialised committees. One of these is the Development Assistance Committee, whose members have agreed to secure an expansion of aggregate volume of resources made available to developing countries and to improve their effectiveness. To this end, members periodically review together both the amount and the nature of their contributions to aid programmes, bilateral and multilateral, and consult each other on all other relevant aspects of their development assistance policies.

The members of the Development Assistance Committee are Australia, Austria, Belgium, Canada, Denmark, Finland, France, Germany, Greece, Ireland, Italy, Japan, Luxembourg, the Netherlands, New Zealand, Norway, Portugal, Spain, Sweden, Switzerland, the United Kingdom, the United States and the Commission of the European Communities.

WORLD HEALTH ORGANIZATION

The World Health Organization was established in 1948 as a specialized agency of the United Nations serving as the directing and coordinating authority for international health matters and public health. One of WHO's constitutional functions is to provide objective and reliable information and advice in the field of human health, a responsibility that it fulfils in part through its extensive programme of publications.

The Organization seeks through its publications to support national health strategies and address the most pressing public health concerns of populations around the world. To respond to the needs of Member States at all levels of development, WHO publishes practical manuals, handbooks and training material for specific categories of health workers; internationally applicable guidelines and standards; reviews and analyses of health policies, programmes and research; and state-of-the-art consensus reports that offer technical advice and recommendations for decision-makers. These books are closely tied to the Organization's priority activities, encompassing disease prevention and control, the development of equitable health systems based on primary health care, and health promotion for individuals and communities. Progress towards better health for all also demands the global dissemination and exchange of information that draws on the knowledge and experience of all WHO's Member countries and the collaboration of world leaders in public health and the biomedical sciences.

To ensure the widest possible availability of authoritative information and guidance on health matters, WHO secures the broad international distribution of its publications and encourages their translation and adaptation. By helping to promote and protect health and prevent and control disease throughout the world, WHO's books contribute to achieving the Organization's principal objective - the attainment by all people of the highest possible level of health.

Publié en français sous le titre :
Pauvreté et santé
Les lignes directrices et ouvrages de référence du CAD

© **Organisation for Economic Co-operation and Development (OECD), World Health Organization (WHO) 2003**
Permission to reproduce or translate all or part of this book should be made to OECD Publications, 2, rue André-Pascal, 75775 Paris Cedex 16, France.

The designations employed and the presentation of the material in this publication do not imply the expression of any opinion whatsoever on the part of the World Health Organization or of the Organisation for Economic Co-operation and Development concerning the legal status of any country, territory, city or area or of its authorities, or concerning the delimitation of its frontiers or boundaries. The World Health Organization and the Organisation for Economic Co-operation and Development do not warrant that the information contained in this publication is complete and correct and shall not be liable for any damages incurred as a result of its use.

WHO Library Cataloguing-in-Publication Data

Poverty and health.

(DAC guidelines and reference series)

1.Poverty 2.Health status 3.Delivery of health care - organization and administration 4.Financing, Health 5.Public policy 6.Intersectoral cooperation 7.Guidelines I.Organisation for Economic Co-operation and Development. Development Assistance Committee.

ISBN 92 4 156236 6 (WHO)   (NLM classification: WA 30)
92 6 410018 0 (OECD)

Foreword

Over recent years OECD and WHO have been collaborating in a range of areas, including on the OECD Health Project which aims to analyse, measure and improve the performance of health systems in OECD countries. This DAC Reference Document dedicated to health and poverty in developing countries is another example of the fruitful collaboration between our two institutions. We have decided to publish it jointly in order to ensure a wide readership in both the development and public health communities.

In developing countries, breaking the vicious circle of poverty and ill health is an essential condition for economic development. The fact that three of the eight Millennium Development Goals are specific to health is evidence of the consensus on this point across the international development community.

In response to this global concern, this Reference Document deepens the approach taken by the DAC Guidelines on Poverty Reduction (2001). It adds further insight into the role of health in reducing poverty and the range of investments required to achieve better health outcomes for poor people as an integral component of poverty reduction strategies.

Achieving better health for poor people requires going well beyond the health sector to take action in related areas such as education, water and sanitation. It also entails looking beyond national programmes to global policies with implications for health, such as trade and the provision of global public goods.

Within the health sector itself, a pro-poor approach is required which includes improving governance, strengthening the delivery and quality of health services, reaching highly vulnerable groups, developing more effective partnerships with the private sector, and designing equitable health financing mechanisms.

However, without significantly increased financing, the poorest countries will remain unable to implement a pro-poor health approach. Urgent action is required to increase ODA to health, which today is less than USD 4 billion per year or about 10% of total ODA. There is also a need to mobilise additional resources from domestic sources, public-private partnerships and philanthropic sources.

This Reference Document was endorsed by the DAC Senior Level Meeting in December 2002. It provides comprehensive, informed and technically robust guidance. We hope it will be used by the donor community, WHO and partner countries to help guide their work on poverty and health.

Secretary-General
Organisation for Economic
Co-operation and Development

Director-General
World Health Organization

Acknowledgements

This DAC Reference Document on Poverty and Health, jointly published by the OECD and WHO, is the result of collective work undertaken by the DAC Network on Poverty Reduction and its Subgroup on Poverty and Health. Over a two-year period, a series of intensive working meetings under the leadership of the POVNET Chair, Claudio Spinedi, and the Subgroup Chair, Wolfgang Bichmann, established the direction of the work and the content of the document.

Senior policy advisers from bilateral aid agencies with expertise in poverty and health, together with representatives of the World Bank, the IMF, UNICEF, UNDP, and UNFPA made significant contributions. Throughout the process, the document benefited from the technical expertise of WHO and particularly from the inputs of John Martin, Rebecca Dodd, and Andrew Cassels.

Membership of the Subgroup was broadened to include the non-governmental sector, and representatives of the Planned Parenthood Foundation and the Aga Khan Development Network made invaluable contributions. In addition, developing country representatives who participated in one meeting made significant oral and written comments.

Thanks are due to staff of the London School of Hygiene and Tropical Medicine, Adrienne Brown from the Institute for Health Sector Development, and particularly to Hilary Standing from the Institute of Development Studies for her extensive inputs and drafting. The document also reflects inputs from a range of officials from OECD directorates, working parties, and networks.

Drawing on the above inputs, the final drafting and editing was done by staff of the Development Co-operation Directorate – Stephanie Baile, Jean Lennock, Paul Isenman and Dag Ehrenpreis, assisted by Julie Seif and Maria Consolati.

Table of Contents

Acronyms

AfDF	African Development Fund
AsDF	Asian Development Fund
AIDS	Acquired Immunodeficiency Syndrome
AKHS	Aga Khan Health Services
AMR	Anti-microbial Resistance
ART	Anti-retroviral Therapy
CMH	Commission on Macroeconomics and Health
CRS	Creditor Reporting System (of the DAC)
DAC	Development Assistance Committee
DHS	Demographic and Health Survey
DOTS	Directly Observed Therapy, Short-Course
DFID	Department for International Development
EC	European Commission
FCTC	Framework Convention on Tobacco Control
GATS	General Agreement on Trade in Services
GAVI	Global Alliance for Vaccines and Immunisation
GFATM	Global Fund for AIDS, Tuberculosis and Malaria
GHI	Global Health Initiatives
GHRF	Global Health Research Fund
GPG	Global Public Good
GTZ*	German Agency for Technical Co-operation
HIV	Human Immunodeficiency Virus
HIPC	Heavily Indebted Poor Countries
IDB Sp F	Inter-American Development Bank, Special Operation Fund
ICRC	International Committee of the Red Cross
ICT	Information and Communications Technology
IDA	International Development Association
IDG	International Development Goal
IHR	International Health Regulations
ILO	International Labour Organization
IMF	International Monetary Fund
LSMS	Living Standards Measurement Survey
MDG	Millennium Development Goal
M&E	Monitoring and Evaluation
MoH	Ministry of Health
MTEF	Medium-Term Expenditure Framework

* Denotes acronym in original language.

NHA	National Health Accounts
NGO	Non-Governmental Organisation
OBA	Output-Based Approaches to Aid
ODA	Official Development Assistance
OECD	Organisation for Economic Co-operation and Development
PPA	Participatory Poverty Assessment
PPP	Public-Private Partnership
PRGF	Poverty Reduction Growth Facility
PRS	Poverty Reduction Strategy
PRSP	Poverty Reduction Strategy Paper
R&D	Research and Development
STD	Sexually-Transmitted Disease
SWAp	Sector-Wide Approach
TB	Tuberculosis
TRIPS	Trade-Related Aspects of Intellectual Property Rights
UN	United Nations
UNAIDS	Joint UN Programme on HIV/AIDS
UNDP	United Nations Development Programme
UN ECOSOC	Economic and Social Council of the United Nations
UNHCR	United Nations High Commission for Refugees
USAID	United States Agency for International Development
WEHAB	Water, Energy, Health, Agriculture and Biodiversity. The WEHAB initiative was proposed by UN Secretary-General Kofi Annan as a contribution to the preparations for the WSSD. It seeks to provide focus and impetus to action in these five key thematic areas.
WHA	World Health Assembly
WHO	World Health Organization
WTO	World Trade Organization

Overview and Purpose

The DAC Reference Document on Poverty and Health, jointly published by the OECD and the World Health Organization (WHO), is the outcome of a joint effort by DAC members working together through the DAC Network on Poverty Reduction. It builds on bilateral agency experience and the work of leading organisations such as the WHO, the World Bank and other United Nations agencies as well as non-governmental organisations. It also draws selectively on the work of the Commission on Macroeconomics and Health, which represents the most systematic and up-to-date review of the evidence linking health to economic development and poverty reduction.

This Reference Document aims to further increase the effectiveness of development co-operation in improving the health of poor people as a means of reducing poverty and achieving the health-related Millennium Development Goals. It expands and deepens the *DAC Guidelines on Poverty Reduction*, which were endorsed by OECD Ministers of Development Co-operation and heads of development agencies at the 2001 DAC High Level Meeting.

This set of policy recommendations is geared to a broad range of development agency staff working in policy and operations, at headquarters and in the field. It provides directions on the most effective ways of supporting a pro-poor health approach in partner countries.

A pro-poor health approach is one that:

- Gives priority to promoting, protecting, and improving the health of the poor (Chapter 1).
- Includes the development of pro-poor health systems, with equitable financing mechanisms (Chapter 2).
- Encompasses policies in areas that disproportionately affect the health of poor people such as education, nutrition, water and sanitation (Chapter 3).
- Is integrated in country-led poverty reduction strategies and health-sector programmes (Chapter 4).
- Takes into account global public goods and policy coherence concerns, including health surveillance, R&D in poverty-related diseases, trade policy issues regarding drugs and vaccines, and migration (Chapter 5).

Key Actions to Promote a Pro-poor Health Approach

PARTNER COUNTRY	ACTION	DEVELOPMENT AGENCY (Support role for partner-led efforts)
1. Demonstrate political will to reduce poverty and achieve the health-related Millennium Development Goals.	**I** **Mobilise political will and additional resources for health**	Encourage greater understanding of the contribution of health to pro-poor growth and development. Foster dialogue on health and other policies that underpin a pro-poor health approach.
2. Mobilise additional domestic resources for health through budget reallocations and HIPC repayment savings. Improve the efficiency of health spending. Improve financial systems for greater transparency and accountability.		Scale up assistance for the achievement of the health-related MDGs and poverty reduction.
3. Assume key public-sector functions in health: policy-making, regulation, purchase and provision of services.	**II** **Develop effective pro-poor health systems**	Strengthen capacity for the execution of the core functions of the ministry of health.
4. Provide accessible, affordable, and responsive quality health services.		Facilitate the identification of disease patterns, and the health service needs of poor people and vulnerable groups.
5. Strengthen health financing systems to allow for equitable access of the poor to health services.		Support capacity in social impact analysis, to make health systems, including financing, more accessible to the poor.
6. Support health policies through decentralisation and greater local capacity to deliver services. Ensure meaningful community participation.		Assist civil society organisations and community representatives to increase their capacity to participate in health policy and programmes.
7. Develop partnerships with the private sector and NGOs for the delivery of health services.		Support strategies to improve service delivery including better public services and partnerships with the private sector to increase coverage.

DAC GUIDELINES AND REFERENCE SERIES: POVERTY AND HEALTH – ISBN 92-64-10018-0 – © OECD, WHO 2003

	PARTNER COUNTRY	ACTION	DEVELOPMENT AGENCY (Support role for partner-led efforts)
8.	Facilitate cross-sectoral collaboration and harmonisation of policy objectives to improve health outcomes. Mandate and resource non-health ministries to do so.	**III** **Focus on other sector policies impacting on poor people's health**	Help generate greater recognition of the potential impact of sector policies on health such as education, nutrition, water and sanitation.
9.	Lead, own and implement a comprehensive health-sector programme and integrate it into the Poverty Reduction Strategy (PRS).	**IV** **Work through country-led poverty reduction strategies and health-sector programmes, and monitor progress towards improved health outcomes**	Promote greater country leadership and ownership for the elaboration and implementation of PRS and health-sector programmes. Work towards common procedures for aid delivery and evaluation.
10.	Improve links and policy consistency between PRS and health-sector programmes (and other sectors impacting on health).		Build capacity for poverty and gender analysis in health.
11.	Ensure that Global Health Initiatives are integrated into national systems.		Ensure that Global Health Initiatives support country ownership and policies.
12.	Select core indicators to monitor health system performance and health outcomes with a focus on equity (including gender), access, quality and financing.		Strengthen national statistical capacity and monitoring systems to measure progress towards health and poverty reduction objectives. Accept a balance between national and international monitoring needs.
13.	Participate in priority-setting for the provision of global public goods (GPGs) for health and integrate it into PRS.	**V** **Promote global public goods and policy coherence for pro-poor health**	Support international initiatives for GPGs for health such as research on affordable drugs and vaccines for diseases of the poor. Integrate support for GPGs in overall development strategies.
14.	Fully explore the potential of TRIPS for providing affordable essential drugs to poor people.		Promote policy coherence – including trade and migration – to support pro-poor health. Follow up the *Doha Declaration on TRIPS and Public Health* regarding affordable access of poor countries to priority drugs and vaccines.

ISBN 92-64-10018-0
DAC Guidelines and Reference Documents
Poverty and Health
© OECD, WHO 2003

Summary

I. Investing in health to reduce poverty

Health is now higher on the international agenda than ever before, and concern for the health of poor people is becoming a central issue in development. Indeed, three of the Millennium Development Goals (MDGs) call for health improvements by 2015: reducing child deaths, maternal mortality, and the spread of HIV/AIDS, malaria and tuberculosis. The nations of the world have agreed that enjoying the highest attainable standard of health is one of the fundamental rights of every human being, without distinction of race, religion, political belief, economic or social condition. *Beyond its intrinsic value to individuals, health is also central to overall human development and to the reduction of poverty.*

- **The poor suffer worse health and die younger.** They have higher than average child and maternal mortality, higher levels of disease, and more limited access to health care and social protection. And gender inequality disadvantages further the health of poor women and girls. *For poor people especially, health is also a crucially important economic asset.* Their livelihoods depend on it. When poor people become ill or injured, the entire household can become trapped in a downward spiral of lost income and high health-care costs. Investment in health is increasingly recognised as an important means of economic development and a prerequisite for developing countries – and particularly for poor people within them – to break out of the cycle of poverty. Good health contributes to development in a number of ways: it increases labour productivity, educational attainment and investment, and it facilitates the demographic transition.

The human and economic rationale for investing in health is mirrored by a growing consensus on the importance of a broad agenda in improving the health of the poor. This Reference Document identifies the essential components of a pro-poor health approach and provides a framework for action within the health system – and beyond it, through policies in other sectors and through global initiatives. Within this framework, the support of development agencies will vary according to the needs, capacities and policies of each partner country.

- **Scaling-up financial resources for health should be a priority.** Without money to buy vaccines and drugs, to build and equip facilities, to ensure adequate staffing, to manage the health system, and to increase investments in other sectors important for health, low-income countries will be unable to meet the health-related MDGs. This requires more financing from the budgets of partner countries as well as substantial increases in external support for health. Development agencies are more likely to mobilise additional resources in support of pro-poor health objectives where: i) there is a clear political will on the part of the partner country to articulate and implement a poverty-reduction strategy and a comprehensive health-sector programme; ii) serious efforts are being made to mobilise domestic resources; iii) there is commitment to manage resources more effectively; and iv) major stakeholders have an opportunity to participate in the planning, management and delivery of interventions. In countries with weak policies, institutions and governance, support to the extent feasible to health and other basic services will be essential to protect the poor and vulnerable – as called for in the DAC work on "difficult partnerships".

II. Supporting pro-poor health systems

A pro-poor health approach gives priority to promoting, protecting and improving the health of poor people. It includes the provision of quality services in public health and personal care, with equitable financing mechanisms, which are essential to improve health and prevent the spiral from ill health to poverty. Development agencies should help partner countries develop pro-poor health systems by strengthening local capacity in several areas.

- **Strengthening the capacity of the public sector to carry out the core functions of policy maker, regulator, purchaser and provider of health services** is central to the development and implementation of pro-poor health systems. Strong institutional and organisational capacity, moreover, is necessary to track the use of resources, and improve human resource strategies. These key issues go beyond the health ministry alone and reflect the necessity of placing health-sector reforms within the context of broader governance reforms.

- **Developing public and private-sector services that are of good quality and responsive to the health needs and demands of poor people is a priority,** necessitating a focus on those diseases – such as malaria, TB, and HIV/AIDS – that affect the poor disproportionately, as well as on reproductive health and non-communicable diseases, such as those linked to tobacco, where the disease burden on the poor is significant. This approach should be complemented by targeting strategies that reach out to poor and vulnerable groups, and by measures that stimulate demand for health services and increase health service accountability to poor communities. To accomplish these objectives, the voices of the poor, as well as those of non-governmental organisations (NGOs) and civil society organisations, must be heard in the planning and implementation process.

- **Better partnership with the private sector is critical.** Poor people make heavy use of private, for-profit and not-for-profit services (NGO and faith-based). The public sector in many developing countries does not have either the capacity to deliver health services itself to the entire population or to ensure that health services delivered by the private sector promote pro-poor health objectives. The type of partnership that governments can develop with private providers will vary according to patterns of use and their relative strengths and qualities. Governments may choose to contract out particular services to NGOs, or seek to improve the quality of services available in the private-for-profit sector. This policy option will require the strengthening of government capacity for regulation, contracting and monitoring.

- **Equitable health financing systems** are an essential part of improving access to health care and protecting the poor from the catastrophic cost of ill health. This goal requires effective social protection strategies, moving towards risk-pooling and prepayment systems and away from out-of-pocket "fee for service" payment for primary health care, which discourages use by poor people.

III. Focusing on key policy areas for pro-poor health

Ensuring that the poor have access to affordable and quality health services is not sufficient in itself to improve the health of the poor. The major determinants of their health depend on actions that lie outside the health sector. To start with, implementing effective pro-poor growth policies as outlined in the DAC *Guidelines on Poverty Reduction* is crucial: without higher incomes, poor people will not be able to afford food or health services. And without growth in revenues, governments will not increase their financing of health services. Other sectoral policies, too, are critically important, especially those for education, food security, safe water, sanitation and energy. The health of the poor can also be improved by reducing their exposure to the risk of addiction to tobacco or alcohol, of road traffic or other injuries, and of the devastating impacts of conflict and natural disasters. Partner governments and development agencies should assess the extent to which policies in key sectors undermine or promote health and broader poverty reduction objectives, prioritise them in terms of importance and the cost-effectiveness of action, and implement appropriate responses. This would include efforts to strengthen capacity related to health objectives within those sectors.

- **Achievement of the three health-related MDGs, for instance, all hinge strongly on reaching the MDGs of gender equality and universal primary education.** Female education, in particular, is strongly linked to improved health care for children, families and communities, and to lower fertility rates. Education is also one of the most effective tools against HIV/AIDS. Conversely, health is a major determinant of educational attainment since it has a direct impact on cognitive abilities and school attendance. There is therefore, a mutual interest in identifying strategies for collaboration both within the formal school system and through non-formal education.

- **Food security and nutrition are critical factors influencing the health of the poor.** Nearly 800 million people in developing countries are chronically hungry. Under-nutrition affects the immune system, increasing the incidence and severity of diseases and is an associated factor in over 50% of all child mortality. Development agencies should focus on improving food security in rural and urban areas through interventions that aim to increase income and access to social services, as well as through targeted maternal and child nutrition programmes.

- **Poor people's health and mortality are directly affected by exposure to environmental threats.** Poor people often live in low-quality urban settlements, or in remote villages on marginal land. There they have limited access to safe water and sanitation, and are exposed to indoor as well as outdoor air pollution. These environmental conditions are a major cause of ill health and death among poor people. The importance of these basic causes of poor health must be integrated into development policies.

IV. Working through country-led strategic frameworks

The commitment to support the health-related MDGs calls for a long-term relationship with partner countries to achieve sustainable health improvements that benefit the poor. Such co-operation should take place within commonly agreed overarching national frameworks that set priorities for policies and programmes.

- **A Poverty Reduction Strategy (PRS), developed and owned by the partner country,** should be the central framework to formulate the broad lines of a pro-poor health approach. It should demonstrate a clear understanding of the causal links between better health and poverty reduction, and include explicit health objectives in the key sectors that influence the health outcomes of poor people. In this way, a PRS can evolve to encourage links between health and policies in other sectors that promote the health of the poor. Since PRSs have limited space for detailed sectoral analysis, they should be supplemented by a more detailed health-sector programme.

- **A health-sector programme is essential** not only for determining and getting needed support within the health sector but also for engaging in a dialogue on the policies and interventions likely to improve the health of poor people. It also provides a national framework for channelling external support. This support may include technical co-operation for capacity building, large projects, sector-wide financing, overall budget support, debt relief and funds from global initiatives. Although having a large number of separate externally funded activities imposes high costs and can distort country priorities, each instrument has advantages and disadvantages. The issue is primarily one of balance, in the context of differing country circumstances.

- **Sector-wide approaches (SWAps) in health merit attention** because they are relatively new and aim to strengthen co-ordination. In SWAps, external partners adhere to the government-led health programme and help support its development through common procedures for management, implementation and, to varying extents, funding. Where SWAps are appropriate, they can help to promote greater local involvement, accountability and capacity in partner countries. The decision to engage in a SWAp in a given country should result from a careful appraisal of policy and institutional conditions. The premise of this kind of partnership is an atmosphere of mutual trust, reduced attribution to any single development agency, and the acceptance of joint accountability and some increase in financial and institutional risk.

- **Partner countries should measure health system performance and health outcomes and the extent to which they are pro-poor.** As part of their efforts to support PRSs and health-sector programmes, development agencies should give priority to strengthening national systems for data collection, monitoring and evaluation and for statistical analysis as these systems are often inadequate in measuring progress towards health and poverty reduction objectives.

V. Promoting policy coherence and global public goods

The health problems of the poor do not stop at national borders. A globalised world presents new risks to health, as is indicated by the rapid spread of HIV/AIDS or the threat of bioterrorism. At the same time, it provides opportunities to prevent, treat or contain disease. Development agencies and partner countries should strengthen ways of working together globally.

- **One way is to promote the development of Global Public Goods for health (GPGs),** which can provide enduring benefits for all countries and all people. This approach includes such actions as medical research and development focused on diseases that most affect the poor, as well as efforts to stem cross-border spread of communicable disease. It is estimated that under 10% of global funding of health research is devoted to diseases or conditions that account for 90% of the global disease burden, and much less than 10% for the problems of poor countries and people. Development agencies have a key role to play in promoting international initiatives to produce new drugs and vaccines, and knowledge focussed on the health problems of the poor. They can provide critical financial resources and help catalyse support for policy coherence and other support within their own countries. Such initiatives include more emphasis on the diseases of low-income countries in the health-research budgets of OECD countries, partnerships with the private sector and civil society to generate funds and expertise for research on these diseases, and consideration of extension of OECD countries' "orphan drug" incentives to the diseases involved.

- **In addition, trade in goods and services and multilateral trade agreements have an increasing influence on the health of the poor.** Of particular significance are those agreements dealing with trade related aspects of intellectual property rights (TRIPS), the General Agreement on Trade in Services (GATS), and trade in hazardous substances. Member agencies should encourage their governments to monitor the implementation of the *Doha Declaration on the TRIPS Agreement and Public Health* from the perspective of the extent to which developing countries can use the TRIPS Agreement for improving their access to those pharmaceutical products important to the health of poor people that are under patent protection. One such issue, which the World Trade Organization Council is considering is that some countries, without their own production capacity, are having problems in making effective use of *compulsory licensing*.

The need for funding for GPGs is largely additional to the need for development agency support of country programmes. The overall increase in external support depends on opportunities for effective use of that support. It also depends on the extent to which public and political support can be mobilised in OECD countries for the propositions set out, in this document and other reports, on the importance and feasibility of helping to improve the health of the poor.

ISBN 92-64-10018-0
DAC Guidelines and Reference Documents
Poverty and Health
© OECD, WHO 2003

Chapter 1

Investing in Health to Reduce Poverty

Abstract. Beyond its intrinsic value to individuals, health is also central to overall human development and poverty reduction. Yet the poor continue to carry a disproportionate burden of ill health. If the health of poor people is to improve, a pro-poor health approach needs to be put in place and supported by development agencies. The nature of that support will be determined by the country context, particularly in the case of "difficult partnerships". Scaling up financial resources for health should be a priority, requiring more financing from the budgets of partner countries as well as substantial increases in external support. In addition, greater commitment on the side of partner countries to improve governance and the poverty focus of policies need to be matched by efforts within development agencies to improve the effectiveness of their assistance.

1. Introduction

Health is now higher on the international agenda than ever before, and concern for the health of poor people is becoming a central issue in development. The nations of the world have agreed that enjoying the highest attainable standard of health is one of the fundamental rights of every human being without distinction of race, religion, political belief and economic or social condition.[1] *Beyond its intrinsic value for individuals, improving and protecting health is also central to overall human development and to the reduction of poverty.* The Millennium Development Goals (MDGs), derived from the UN Millennium Declaration, commit countries to halving extreme income poverty and to achieving improvements in health by 2015.[2] Three of the eight goals are health-related, calling for a two-thirds reduction in child mortality, a three-quarters reduction in maternal mortality, and a halt to the spread of HIV/AIDS, malaria and tuberculosis. In addition the eighth goal, re. developing a global partnership for development, calls for developing countries to have access to affordable essential drugs. Although each goal contributes in itself to the overall aim of poverty reduction, an essential message is that they are interdependent.

2. Poverty and health

The poor suffer worse health and die younger. They have higher than average child and maternal mortality, higher levels of disease, more limited access to health care and social protection, and gender inequality disadvantages further the health of poor women and girls. For poor people especially, health is also a crucially important economic asset. Their livelihoods depend on it. When a poor or socially vulnerable person becomes ill or injured, the entire household can become trapped in a downward spiral of lost income and high health care costs. The cascading effects may include diverting time from generating an income or from schooling to care for the sick; they may also force the sale of assets required for livelihoods. Poor people are more vulnerable to this downward spiral as they are more prone to disease and have more limited access to health care and social insurance.

The *DAC Guidelines on Poverty Reduction* present a practical definition of poverty, placing it in a broader framework of causes and appropriate policy actions. *The five core dimensions of poverty reflect the deprivation of human capabilities*: economic (income, livelihoods, decent work), human (health, education), political (empowerment, rights, voice), socio-cultural (status, dignity) and protective (insecurity, risk, vulnerability). Measures to promote gender equality and to protect the environment are essential for reducing poverty in all these dimensions. The DAC Guidelines emphasise that some social categories are particularly affected by severe poverty, among them indigenous populations, minority and socially excluded groups, refugees or displaced persons, the mentally or physically disabled and people living with HIV/AIDS. These groups are among the poorest of the poor in many societies and require special attention in policy action for poverty reduction.

DAC GUIDELINES AND REFERENCE SERIES: POVERTY AND HEALTH – ISBN 92-64-10018-0 – © OECD, WHO 2003

Gender inequality is a major determinant of poverty and ill health. Poor women and girls are worse off, in relation to assets and entitlements, within the household and in society. Socio-cultural beliefs about the roles of men and women contribute to this inequality. Poor women and girls may experience even deeper disadvantage in access to resources for health, such as cash and financing schemes, services, and "voice". Some categories of women and children are especially vulnerable – for example elderly widows, unsupported female- and child-headed households, and street children. Women are also major producers of health care through their roles as household managers and carers. But the health, including the reproductive health, of poor women and girls suffers from inadequate nutrition, heavy workloads and neglect of basic health care, factors aggravated by exposure to sexual abuse and interpersonal violence. All have a serious effect on human development and the formation of human capital. Action on gender inequalities is therefore an essential element of a pro-poor approach to health.

3. The economic rationale for investing in the health of the poor

Investment in health is also increasingly recognised as an important – and previously under-estimated – means of economic development. As the Commission on Macroeconomics and Health (CMH) of the World Health Organization (WHO) has shown, substantially improved health outcomes are a prerequisite if developing countries are to break out of the circle of poverty.[3] Good health contributes to development through a number of pathways, which partly overlap but in each case add to the total impact:

- **Higher labour productivity.** Healthier workers are more productive, earn higher wages, and miss fewer days of work than those who are ill. This increases output, reduces turnover in the workforce, and increases enterprise profitability and agricultural production.

- **Higher rates of domestic and foreign investment.** Increased labour productivity in turn creates incentives for investment. In addition, controlling endemic and epidemic diseases, such as HIV/AIDS, is likely to encourage foreign investment, both by increasing growth opportunities for them and by reducing health risks for their personnel.

- **Improved human capital.** Healthy children have better cognitive potential. As health improves, rates of absenteeism and early school drop-outs fall, and children learn better, leading to growth in the human capital base.

- **Higher rates of national savings.** Healthy people have more resources to devote to savings, and people who live longer save for retirement. These savings in turn provide funds for capital investment.

- **Demographic changes.** Improvements in both health and education contribute to lower rates of fertility and mortality. After a delay, fertility falls faster than mortality, slowing population growth and reducing the "dependency ratio" (the ratio of active workers to dependants). This "demographic dividend" has been shown to be an important source of growth in per capita income for low-income countries.[4]

In addition to their beneficial macro-economic impact, *health improvements have inter-generational spill-over effects* that are clearly shown in micro-economic activities, not least in the household itself. The "demographic dividend" is particularly important for the poor as they tend to have more children, and less to "invest" in the education and health of each child. With the spread of better health care and education, family size declines. Children are more likely to escape the cognitive and physical consequences of childhood diseases and to do better in school. These children are less likely to suffer disability and impairment in later life and so are less likely to face catastrophic medical expenses and more likely to achieve their earning potential. Then, as healthy adults, they have more resources to invest in the care, health and education of their own children.

4. Defining a pro-poor health approach

The broad development impact of health investment points to the importance of a comprehensive approach to improving the health of poor people. Although the technical knowledge to address the main causes of ill-health already exists, the poor continue to carry a disproportionate burden of disease. If the health of poor people is to improve, the following key elements of a pro-poor approach must be in place, and priorities for development co-operation identified in this context.

What is a pro-poor health approach?

A pro-poor health approach is one that gives priority to promoting, protecting and improving the health of the poor. It includes the provision of quality public health and personal care services, with equitable financing mechanisms. It goes beyond the health sector to encompass policies in areas that affect the health of the poor disproportionately, such as education, nutrition, water and sanitation. Finally, it is concerned with global action on the effects of trade in health services, intellectual property rights, and the funding of health research as they impact on the health of the poor in developing countries.

A pro-poor health approach builds on the following four pillars.

- **Health systems** comprise the promotive, preventive, curative and rehabilitative services delivered by health personnel and their support structures (*e.g.* drug-procurement systems). They include both public- and private-sector services (for-profit and not-for-profit), formal and informal, as well as traditional services, and home- and family-based care. In many developing countries health systems are weak and fragmented, with the result that millions of the world's poor do not have access to the public health services and personal care they need. In this respect, a major challenge is to address the gender, ethnic and socio-economic biases in health service delivery in order to reach vulnerable groups and groups with special needs.

- **Health financing and broader social protection** strategies are necessary to protect the poor and socially vulnerable from the impoverishing costs of health care. This requires increasing the pooling of risk, cross-subsidy and protection against health shocks, in the context of a comprehensive review of the social protection of the poor.

- **Key policy areas beyond the health sector.** The health of poor people, in particular, is determined by a wide range of factors, including income, education level, food security, environmental conditions, and access to water and sanitation. Economic, trade and fiscal policies are also important determinants of household incomes and nutritional status. They have an impact on inequality and exclusion, whether by gender, ethnicity or socio-economic groups, and these in turn have a major impact on health status. It is therefore necessary to assess the health impact of policies and activities whose primary purpose is not health but which may affect, beneficial or adverse, health outcomes; and

DAC GUIDELINES AND REFERENCE SERIES: POVERTY AND HEALTH – ISBN 92-64-10018-0 – © OECD, WHO 2003

action will be required to optimise the positive impacts and eliminate or reduce those that are undesired. National Poverty Reduction Strategies (PRS) provide an important framework to connect policies outside the health sector with pro-poor health objectives.

- **Promoting policy coherence and global public goods.** A globalised world presents new risks to health, as is indicated by the rapid spread of HIV/AIDS or the threat of bioterrorism. At the same time, it provides opportunities to prevent, treat or contain diseases. International action – such as provision of global public goods, multilateral agreements on trade and investment, and environmental conventions – should complement other pro-poor health strategies.

5. The role of development co-operation in different country contexts

The ways in which development agencies can support a pro-poor health approach should be determined by the specific context of each partner country. Development agencies should consider the different kinds of transition occurring in partner countries and associated economic, social and political factors influencing pro-poor health interventions. The following broad typology of countries, adapted from OECD/DAC work on "difficult partnerships", suggests how country contexts can influence the type of support an agency may propose.

- **Non-aid-dependent countries.** These include middle-income countries where systems of public or private social security and health care are established or becoming so, but with uneven performance by their health systems and unmet health needs. They also include transition countries moving from central planning to a market economy. Both groups include countries with pluralistic health systems with high degrees of private provision. These countries are often, however, facing substantial problems of poverty and inequality. In health, as in other sectors, the role of development co-operation in these countries is modest financially, but often important in facilitating new approaches and innovations. An example is assistance in improving strategies or strengthening the capacity to direct health resources to poor and vulnerable groups.

- **Low-income countries with relatively good poverty reduction and pro-poor social-sector strategies but limited capacity to implement the desired changes.** These are countries with a policy environment and government commitment conducive to improving equity in health systems performance and strengthening the governance and accountability of social sectors. They receive substantial amounts of official development assistance (ODA) which, in the health sector, will be in the form of a mix of budget support, sector programming and project funding. Key areas for assistance may include support for systemic reforms in pro-poor financing, human resources, targeting and social protection, as well as contracting with different types of providers. They also include support for initiatives involving civil society and poorer citizens in consultation, planning, managing or monitoring health service delivery.

- **Low-income countries uncommitted to, or still in early stages of developing poverty reduction and pro-poor social-sector strategies and lacking institutional capacity.** These countries are most often involved in or recovering from large-scale violent conflict. These include collapsed states with few or no functioning institutions (not least markets) and little or no organised health care provision, as well as countries where earlier capacity has been seriously damaged. They suffer from weak governance and decayed public health systems. Poor people frequently resort to traditional medicine and often have no access to reasonable quality medical care. Provision of health care of reasonable quality is typically provided by NGOs, in limited areas of coverage. Areas for development assistance include support for trying out different models of service provision involving non-state providers (particularly but not exclusively NGOs), as well as local governments that have reasonable capacity. It is important, though, to recognise that these "parallel structures" have real costs in the building of sustainable institutional solutions. Agencies can help strengthen demand-side initiatives such as involvement by user groups and civil society, and improve basic monitoring capacity for pro-poor health indicators. It is also important to find ways to repair and restore basic services in water and sanitation. There may be opportunities for agencies to support extension of vaccination and other selected basic services even in areas more or less completely deprived of health care. This can occur even in the midst of conflict, with "Days of Tranquillity" in which civil society is mobilised to provide these services during temporary truces.

- **Countries with weak commitment and/or capacity but where there is more scope for improving development co-operation partnerships.** In these countries, development co-operation would be primarily via project assistance. There would be substantial, but less, reliance on parallel delivery structures and more efforts to assist in capacity development for public-sector provision and regulatory functions.

6. Mobilising resources for pro-poor health

As stated above, improving the health of the poor is an investment in economic growth and development and should be a priority for reducing poverty. The lack of resources allocated to health is not the only obstacle to the effective implementation of pro-poor health policies, but it is a major, and inescapable, part of the problem. A minimally adequate set of interventions and the infrastructure necessary to deliver them is estimated to cost in the order of USD 30 to 40 per capita to meet the basic health needs of the poor.[5] In 2000, the WHO calculated a figure of USD 60 per capita for a more comprehensive health system.[6] This compares with an average level of health expenditures in the Least Developed Countries of USD 11 per year. Current spending, much of which is not for the poor, falls far short of the minimum to meet basic needs. Without money to buy vaccines and drugs, to build and equip facilities, to ensure adequate staffing and to manage the health system, governments in low- and middle-income countries will be unable to make progress in improving the health of the poor.

- **Increased resources should come from a combination of public, private, domestic and external sources, including ODA and Global Health Initiatives (GHIs).** Some increases in government spending for health are possible in most partner countries. National health budgets should reflect the urgency of the poverty and health challenge, both in terms of the size of the budget for health and other social sectors, and the share of health resources allocated to the activities likely to benefit the poorest groups. A number of countries are aiming to increase the share of resources allocated to primary health care, including through channelling savings from debt relief under the Highly Indebted Poor Countries initiative (HIPC) into health. In many partner countries, the distribution of resources benefits highly advanced services at the expense of primary health care and district hospital services. Development agencies should engage in a constructive dialogue to encourage an allocation of resources that benefits the poor and socially vulnerable. In almost all cases, though, the resources released through such means will be limited relative to health needs. The poorest countries will remain unable to provide sufficient resources to meet pro-poor health objectives without significantly increased external financing.

Table 1. **Official development assistance (ODA) to health, 1996-2001: annual average commitment and share in total aid allocated by sector**

	USD million		% of Donor Total		Donors share of Total ODA to Health	
	1996-98	1999-01	1996-98	1999-01	1996-98	1999-01
Australia	83	124	11	17	2	3
Austria	23	55	11	21	1	2
Belgium	56	66	19	19	2	2
Canada	36	69	6	13	1	2
Denmark	90	56	13	10	3	2
Finland	13	17	8	11	0	0
France	100	59	5	5	3	2
Germany	163	125	7	5	5	3
Italy	26	38	10	12	1	1
Japan	242	152	2	2	7	4
Netherlands	140	145	11	13	4	4
Norway	42	92	10	13	1	3
Portugal	..	7	..	5	..	0
Spain	117	92	22	13	4	3
Sweden	73	73	10	13	2	2
Switzerland	30	34	9	8	1	1
United Kingdom	233	500	16	21	7	14
United States	733	1 108	25	18	22	30
TOTAL DAC	**2 201**	**2 817**	**9**	**11**	**66**	**77**
AfDF	59	66	11	9	2	2
AsDF	45	75	3	7	1	2
EC	83	162	8	9	3	4
IDA	893	529	16	9	27	14
IDB Sp F	42	16	8	5	1	1
TOTAL MULTILATERAL	**1 122**	**848**	**12**	**9**	**34**	**23**
GRAND TOTAL	**3 323**	**3 665**	**10**	**10**	**100**	**100**

Notes: ODA to health includes reproductive health. Greece, Luxembourg and New Zealand do not report to the OECD Creditor Reporting System (CRS) and Ireland reports since 2000 only. Annual DAC statistics show an average commitment of USD 4 million in 1999-2001 (6% of its total), USD 11 million (24%), USD 4 million (7%) and USD 22 million (21%) for Greece, Luxembourg, New Zealand and Ireland respectively. Approximately 65-70% of DAC members' bilateral ODA can be allocated by sector. Contributions not susceptible to allocation by sector (*e.g.* structural adjustment, balance-of-payments support, debt-related initiatives, and emergency assistance) are excluded from the denominator in order to better reflect the sectoral focus of development agencies' programmes.

Excluded from the OECD figures is bilateral support for UN agencies such as WHO and UNICEF and aid flows at non-concessional terms. Estimates prepared for the CMH put total development assistance to health (including these categories and flows from non-profit foundations) at USD 6.7 billion a year in the late 1990s. See WHO (2001).

Source: OECD.

Total aid commitments from DAC members to health provided through bilateral and multilateral channels has averaged close to USD 3.7 billion per year for 1999-2001. As shown in Table 1, aid to health as a share of ODA has remained at a level of 10% in recent years. The current allocations are far below the estimated funding needs in the sector.

- **Development agencies are more likely to mobilise resources in support of pro-poor health objectives where:** i) there is a clear political will on the part of the partner country to articulate and implement a poverty reduction strategy and a closely-linked health-sector programme; ii) serious efforts are being made to mobilise domestic resources; iii) there is commitment to manage resources more effectively; and iv) major civil-society stakeholders have an opportunity to participate in the planning, management and delivery of interventions. The differing situation of "difficult partnerships", where there are few opportunities to raise additional domestic resources, has been discussed above.

7. Improving the effectiveness of development co-operation

Development agencies should consider how to improve their own capacity to support pro-poor health objectives and overcome the constraints that limit the effectiveness of development co-operation, with special emphasis on:

- **Capacity building and broader concerns of governance**. Support for effective national health systems is critical to shift more responsibility to partner countries to design and implement their health policies and programmes. Capacity building should go beyond the health sector. It requires viewing pro-poor health approaches in a larger context of political and economic restructuring, fiscal policy, administrative reform and the strengthening of participation and democratic systems. ODA should play a catalytic role in all these areas if investments in health and poverty reduction are to be sustainable.

- **Policy dialogue is an integral element of development co-operation.** It does not involve direct transfer of resources, and yet it is essential to forge stronger partnerships around shared objectives and to elevate pro-poor health objectives to the top of the political agenda. Since improving health outcomes require a multi-sectoral approach, policy dialogue must be extended to involve other ministries (primarily those dealing with water, sanitation, nutrition, transport and energy) taking into account the macro-economic and cross-sectoral implications of pro-poor health objectives.

- **Co-ordination is essential** in order to mobilise and concentrate resources on the MDGs and pro-poor health objectives. The co-ordination of external partners, led by government, magnifies the effectiveness of development co-operation programmes not least because it encourages development agencies to reinforce and complement their programmes in support of the objectives specified in the poverty reduction strategy (PRS) and the health-sector plan.

- **Programme support is particularly effective in addressing sector-wide issues** and in implementing comprehensive inter-sectoral plans such as those required for pro-poor health. It is, however, limited to partner countries with a strong commitment to pro-poor health and transparent financial management and reporting systems. The harmonisation of development agency procedures in this context can help lower transaction costs and reduce the burden on partner countries of having to comply with multiple, and often differing, requirements. In other countries, development agencies should work through a combination of aid instruments which fit national conditions.

- **Monitoring and evaluation.** In order to secure long-term commitment from development agencies and mobilise additional resources, special emphasis should be given to monitoring health system performance and health outcomes and the extent to which they are pro-poor.

Notes

1. Constitution of the World Health Organization (1948).

2. See Table 2 in Chapter 4 for the health related MDGs. The other goals are to eradicate extreme poverty and hunger, to achieve universal primary education, to promote gender equality and empower women, and to ensure environmental sustainability.

3. WHO (2001), *Macroeconomics and Health: Investing in Health for Economic Development, Report of the Commission on Macroeconomics and Health*, WHO, Geneva.

4. However, low and middle-income countries with high rates of HIV/AIDS have high death rates among those of working age, which increases the dependency ratio and reduces growth. In contrast, higher-income countries have little room for the birth rate to decline further and a growing number of retirees; so their dependency ratios are increasing. See Birdsall, N., A.C. Kelley and S. Sinding (eds.) (2001), *Population Matters: Demographic Change, Economic Growth, and Poverty in the Developing World*, Oxford University Press, New York.

5. This figure does not include important elements such as family planning, tertiary hospitals and emergencies, which would also need to be part of any operational health system. WHO (2001), *op. cit.*

6. WHO (2000), *The World Health Report 2000: Health Systems: Improving Performance*, WHO, Geneva.

ISBN 92-64-10018-0
DAC Guidelines and Reference Documents
Poverty and Health
© OECD, WHO 2003

Chapter 2

Supporting Pro-poor Health Systems

Abstract. *Development agencies are committed to working in partnership with developing countries to develop health systems that provide quality public health programmes and personal (i.e. individual) health services that are accessible by the poor and nearly poor. This can be achieved in four complementary ways. First, by strengthening government capacity to steward the health sector in order to improve the design and implementation of pro-poor health policies. Second, by strengthening the poverty focus of health system delivery, responding better to the needs of the poorest and most vulnerable, partly through increasing their participation. Third, by helping countries manage a pluralistic health system, with more effective roles for the public sector, the private for-profit sector, and the not-for-profit sector, all of which have roles in improving access and quality. Finally, by supporting a move towards more equitable health financing mechanisms based on pre-payment and risk pooling.*

1. Introduction

Health systems comprise promotion, prevention, curative and rehabilitation services delivered by health workers and related support structures (*e.g.* drug procurement systems). They include both public services, private for-profit and not-for-profit (NGO, including those that are faith-based) services, formal and informal services, as well as traditional health care, and home/family-based care. A health system also includes other related activities, such as medical research and development. In many developing countries health services are often ineffective, with the result that hundreds of millions of the world's poor do not have access to the public health and personal care they need. Ensuring that people have access to effective and affordable health services is not only vital to give them opportunities to improve their lives but is an essential measure of social protection to prevent the spiral from ill health to poverty.

As shown in Figure 1, the current allocation of ODA to health covers all aspects of health systems from basic health care to medical services, training, and research. Bilateral and multilateral development assistance has broadly the same emphasis except for health policy and management, which receives a greater proportion of multilateral funding.

Figure 1. **Sub-sectoral breakdown of ODA to health, 1999-2001**

Inner: bilateral assistance, Outer: all ODA

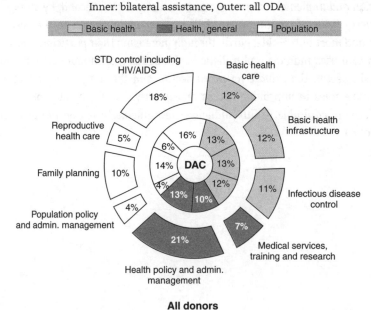

Source: OECD.

DAC GUIDELINES AND REFERENCE DOCUMENTS: POVERTY AND HEALTH – ISBN 92-64-10018-0 – © OECD, WHO 2003

2. Health-sector stewardship

Developing country governments and, specifically, ministries of health are responsible for the performance of the health sector and the extent to which it meets pro-poor objectives. In many countries, *the role of government in the provision of health care is being redefined: the focus is now more on its stewardship functions of policy maker, regulator and purchaser, and not only as service provider.* Effective health-sector stewardship – steering, supervising and enforcing the implementation of health policies and strategies – is of central importance to a pro-poor health system. It requires clear systems to support, communicate and manage relationships, whether between public and private groups or between central, regional and district authorities. One key element is the closer tracking of expenditure and the reduction of "leakage" from the system so as to improve the efficiency and equity of resource allocation and health system performance in general and for the poor in particular. This requires the wider use of such tools as national health accounts and public expenditure tracking surveys.

Strong capacity in partner governments is an essential, though not a sufficient, condition for improving the pro-poor focus of health policies, services and financing. Yet in many developing countries, the capacity to execute these multiple functions is limited and stewardship weak. Moreover, the effectiveness of these functions depends on the context in which they are performed, and a range of factors – such as per capita income, the degrees of poverty and of inequality, political legitimacy, and instability caused by conflict – can have a major influence. The extent of collaboration and co-ordination with other parts of government (such as ministries of planning and finance and those in charge of civil service reform and management) are also critical determinants. Finally, the extent to which the principles of good governance – transparency, accountability, participation, rule of law, and equity – guide the execution of these functions is another central consideration.

Development agencies can play a vital role in strengthening the capacity of partner governments provided that they take into account the impact of political and institutional factors. In the most highly constrained countries with deficient government, weak rule of law, corruption or previous or continuing conflict, the ability to perform any of these functions will be even more limited. In these countries, the urgent health needs of the poor should be met through special strategies (see Section 3.1) while measures to strengthen the capacity of ministries of health, particularly at their lower tiers and in decentralised management, through education, training, and management strengthening, should not be neglected.

2.1. Policy-making in the health sector

Health policy in partner countries is formulated in complex political and economic environments. Development agencies can play a supportive role in ensuring that policies have an explicit focus on pro-poor health objectives and are formulated in consultation with a broad range of stakeholders across government and civil society, including the poor themselves. Health policies should clearly identify the roles that all health actors – including NGOs, community-based organisations and the private-for-profit sector – have to play in improving health outcomes for poor people. Partner countries' planning and health ministries and development agencies, moreover, should take concerted action to ensure that the importance of health is recognised across government as central to reducing poverty and attaining broader development objectives, and that this goal is reflected in poverty reduction strategies.

2.2. The regulatory role of government

Development agencies have varying perspectives on the ideal mix of public- and private-sector participation in health service delivery in developing countries, perspectives which are often related to the public-private mix of the health system in their own country. Nonetheless, the reality of extensive use of private health services by the poor in partner countries, combined with limited capacity to expand government services, has led to an increased emphasis on how to ensure that public priorities are met regardless of who delivers the services.

One important way of meeting public priorities is through a *regulatory role* which aims to improve overall governance and the delivery and quality of health services – in the public, private and NGO sectors – while protecting the poor from excessive or unaffordable health care costs. Although regulation should be regarded as a positive role of government well beyond the health sector, in many countries it is interpreted negatively and has been strongly associated with corruption. Yet regulation means more than ensuring compliance: it involves guidelines for the implementation of health policies, including professional certification and supervision of health personnel, as well as policies on the quality and availability of drugs. The setting of standards for health service providers and ensuring an adequate quality of care can have a substantial impact on the take-up of health services, particularly by poor people. In many partner countries, regulation is generally weak both in design (many activities lack an appropriate structure of regulation and policy) and implementation (regulations are not enforced).

Governments can help foster pro-poor health objectives by developing partnerships with non-state health actors – for-profit and not-for-profit – and using appropriate regulation, which should ensure that private provision complements public provision and helps achieve national priorities. This goal requires a better understanding of how poor people use private-sector services, including in the informal private sector. But where government is unable to design and enforce such regulation, development agencies should provide assistance in ways that both improve the delivery of health services in the short term and also help to develop longer-term strategies to increase the regulatory capacity of government as a whole.

2.3. The role of government as purchaser of services

As a result of limited government delivery capacity, increased attention is being given to the role of government in purchasing health services – paying providers to deliver a specified or unspecified set of health interventions. Recently an active role in purchasing started to be introduced into several government health systems (see Section 4). Provided that there are pro-poor benchmarks in contracts and monitoring, purchasing services from the private sector, particularly from NGOs and faith-based service providers, can improve delivery to poor and vulnerable groups that are currently under-served.

2.4. The role of government as service provider

When governments provide health services themselves, they face considerable challenges in meeting pro-poor health objectives. They have to focus on how to improve health systems so that the services they provide address the principal health requirements of poor people, reach vulnerable groups more effectively, and improve their health. Other complex issues – such as improving drug supply, procurement and logistics, upgrading national and local management information systems, and using quality assurance methods to improve the quality of the services provided – have remained unresolved and warrant further support for the improvement of managerial and technical capacity. Since the quality of service provision is highly dependent on the availability and skills of health professionals, the following section considers human resource strategies in more detail.

Focusing on human resource strategies

Partner countries typically face a shortage of key health professionals, unsupervised personnel, high attrition rates, low government salaries supplemented by informal cash payments, and sometimes conflicts of interest between private- and public-sector employment. In many countries, health workers are themselves poor which contributes to a demoralised workforce offering a poor quality of service. As a result, *a major part of the workforce is ill equipped, and ill supported to meet the health challenge* that lies before them. Health ministries face many obstacles to the development of effective human resource policies. These include weak or inflexible civil service policy, including staff remaining unpaid or "ghost workers" who get paid but rarely or never work; limited autonomy and budget for the health sector to train and allocate staff; loss of staff to higher-paid jobs overseas or in the private sector; geographical imbalances in the distribution of the workforce; and the impact of illness and premature death because of HIV/AIDS.

Development agencies can play a major role in improving the focus on human resource strategies, which are integrated into health sector and wider civil service reforms. Ways in which they can assist include support to partner efforts to:

- **Analyse the mix of personnel and skills** required to deliver expanded services effectively. For example, expanding the numbers of nurses, midwives and trained medical assistants and reviewing their responsibilities may be more appropriate than increasing the numbers of doctors.

- **Reorient training** from service-based curricula with a strong curative bias towards a more holistic approach that includes preventive as well as promotive sciences.

- **Address pay and non-pay incentives** including adequate pay for health workers and decent accommodation, protection from violence, improving personal safety (particularly for women staff), in-service learning and supportive supervision. This will often call attention to, and may require, broader civil-service reform.

- **Improve job opportunities, pay and conditions** to attract health workers, especially women, to remote, under-served areas where the majority of poor people live and where the quantity and quality of services available is inadequate.[1] These strategies should take account of the way in which deployment and incentives are affected by gender.

- **Improve and expand the use of information and communications technology (ICT)** in the training and education programmes undertaken by health service personnel. This would help address such problems as poor standards in training, limited continuing education, and lack of access to up-to-date information and techniques; it could also reduce the heavy burden that the collection of data imposes on health facilities.[2]

In summary, development agencies should take a strategic approach to strengthen the capacity of governments in the health sector to fulfil their multiple functions as policy maker, regulator, purchaser and service provider. This may include a combination of training, formal education, secondments, institutional twinning, technology transfer, the creation of an open environment for change, and improvements in communication among staff and between organisations and services.[3]

3. Strengthening the delivery of health services

3.1. Addressing the priority health needs of the poor

The burden of communicable and non-communicable diseases

Communicable diseases – particularly those associated with a poor environment or maternal, perinatal and nutritional problems – account for most instances of ill health in low-income countries and among the poor in middle-income countries. Acute respiratory infection, diarrhoea, malaria and measles are responsible for most childhood mortality and morbidity. Malaria causes the deaths of one million people each year and tuberculosis some two million. HIV/AIDS is an increasing cause of premature death across sub-Saharan Africa and Asia (see Box 1).

Non-communicable diseases – such as diabetes, cardiovascular disease, respiratory problems caused by air pollution, psychosocial problems and injuries from road-traffic crashes and interpersonal violence (see Chapter 3) – also have a marked impact on the health of poor populations.[4] Tobacco-related diseases are strongly related to poverty. Habitual tobacco use is projected to cause an estimated seven million additional deaths annually from these diseases by 2030 in developing countries, 50% of them in Asia (see Box 2).[5] As more developing countries complete the demographic transition, non-communicable diseases will increase in importance, with many countries suffering the double burden of high rates of both communicable and non-communicable diseases.

The reproductive health challenge

Poor maternal health, sexually transmitted diseases and limited access to family planning services put a sizeable burden of ill health upon poor women. *Reducing maternal mortality and morbidity is a major challenge* – and the MDGs include a targeted reduction by three-quarters in the maternal mortality ratio by 2015. On average, one woman dies every minute from complications during pregnancy or in childbirth. Maternal mortality, like child mortality, provides a telling proxy for the effects of poverty, gender inequality and lack of accessible health services.[6] More than 99% of the estimated 585 000 deaths annually during pregnancy or in childbirth occur in developing countries, and 90% in sub-Saharan Africa.[7] At least 13% of these deaths are related to the 46 million abortions that take place every year.[8] In addition to the high risk of death, an estimated 300 million women currently live with health problems or disabilities resulting from pregnancy.[9] Of these, between 15 million and 20 million develop severe incapacitating disabilities.[10]

Although there has been some increase in the percentage of women who have been able to rely on skilled attendance when they gave birth, programmes have generally failed to focus on the most cost-effective interventions, such as basic antenatal, delivery and post-partum care.[11] Successful programmes depend particularly on the effectiveness of health systems, including improved referral. Indeed, strengthening health services to reduce maternal mortality would ensure they are also capable of addressing a range of other health priorities. Development agencies should provide better support for measures that increase access to maternal health services, including health system strengthening

Box 1. **HIV/AIDS: a development problem**

HIV/AIDS now threatens previous achievements in health: it has already caused 25 million deaths worldwide. Forty-two million people are currently infected with the virus, 29.4 million of them in sub-Saharan Africa, and most are likely to die prematurely from AIDS-related conditions. HIV/AIDS usually affects adults in their prime income-generating or child-bearing years. HIV/AIDS has an impoverishing impact on households, can drive the near poor into poverty, and be devastating for the poorest groups – and poverty and gender inequality make people more vulnerable to infection.[1]

The extent of the HIV epidemic has led to an unprecedented demand for health services in the worst-affected countries at the same time as it eroded the capacity of health workers to respond to the increased demand. Yet an efficient health service is fundamental to an effective response to the disease. Among the essential health-sector interventions that will reduce the spread and impact of HIV are improved diagnosis and treatment of sexually transmitted diseases (STDs), voluntary counselling and testing, access to treatment for opportunistic infections, interventions to reduce mother-to-child transmission, access to condoms, improved home-based care and counselling, and access to anti-retroviral therapy (ART).

NGOs, for-profit organisations and large employers are increasingly providing ART, particularly in urban areas. In public health systems of most low-income countries, by contrast, capacity is inadequate and substantial improvements will be required in infrastructure, in human resources, and in the ability to maintain an uninterrupted supply of drugs before wider access to ART can be implemented. It is widely expected that more effective care, as well as research results that are reducing the complexity of ART, will boost the effectiveness of HIV-prevention programmes. Yet there is continuing discussion about the extent to which negative externalities may emerge. Development agencies and partner governments must address several issues: the risk that safer-sex messages may be ignored if the consequences of infection are downplayed; the threat of widespread drug-resistance; and the extent of financing available for ART without cutting back on resources for HIV/AIDS control programmes and other essential health interventions. On the financing issue, though, it is important to distinguish between *ex ante* needs for external financing, taking account of ART that can be successfully administered, and *ex post* allocation of limited funds available.

Since most experience of ART has been gained in resource-rich, industrialised countries, development agencies can play an important role by supporting particular research activities, not least clinical trials relevant to resource-limited settings, the capacity of health systems to deliver and monitor treatment, or the impact of access to ART on sexual behaviour.[2]

In addition, actions outside the health sector are crucial and can have a major impact on HIV/AIDS prevention. Ministries of finance, education, agriculture, youth and planning, among others, should be involved in developing and implementing the HIV/AIDS response, and HIV/AIDS prevention should feature prominently in poverty reduction strategies.

1. A study of Burkina Faso, Rwanda, and Uganda calculated that AIDS will increase the percentage of people living in extreme poverty from 45% in 2000 to 51% in 2015. UNAIDS Fact Sheet (2002) Accessible at www.unaids.org/worldaidsday/2002/press/index.html#facts
2. WHO (2002), *Scaling Up Anti-Retroviral Therapy in Resource-Limited Settings: A Public Health Approach.* WHO, Geneva.

Box 2. **Tobacco, alcohol and drug abuse:
preventable causes of poverty and ill health**

Tobacco, alcohol and drug abuse are widespread – but preventable – causes of death and disability. Every year approximately four million people worldwide die as a result of tobacco-related illnesses, half of these in developing countries. The 900 million smokers living in developing countries account for 70% of global tobacco consumption. Tobacco use has a profound effect on poverty and malnutrition in low-income countries, when poor families purchase addictive tobacco rather than food. There are grave poverty implications of the high prevalence of tobacco use among men with low education and low incomes, which raises substantially the risks they run of serious diseases and premature death.

Policies and interventions to help smokers quit, and to discourage others from starting, are an important part of national and international efforts to improve the health and well-being of poor people. Development agencies should use policy dialogue and technical and financial co-operation to support policy change. The most important are raising taxes on tobacco,[1] bans (or, where this is not acceptable, sharp restrictions) on cigarette advertising and promotion, increased access to nicotine-replacement therapies, and restrictions on exposure to second-hand smoke. These policy changes are already under way, to varying extents, in all DAC member countries.

Alcohol-related diseases affect 5 to 10% of the world's population each year and alcohol use is the fourth-highest cause of disability worldwide. Alcohol consumption is rising in many developing countries and in sub-Saharan Africa it is a major factor in deaths from injury.[2] Drug abuse is also a major cause of ill health and social problems. The use of scarce financial resources to buy alcohol and narcotics carries implications for household economic security and an increased risk of poverty beyond its direct impact on health status.

1. Studies show that for every 10% increase in prices via increased taxation, tobacco consumption goes down by about 5 to 8% – with poorer countries, and people, at the upper end of that range. Tobacco smuggling reduces this impact, but it still remains highly significant. [See WHO (2002), *Improving Health Outcomes of the Poor*, The Report of Working Group 5 of the Commission on Macroeconomics and Health, WHO, Geneva.]
2. Murray, C.J.L. and A.D. Lopez (1996), *The global burden of disease*, Cambridge, MA: Harvard University Press. Reproduced in "Deaths among men, attributable to and averted by alcohol, 1990", *British Medical Journal (BMJ)* 2002; 325: 964.

and increased access to antenatal care, skilled care during labour and delivery, and access to emergency obstetric care in district hospitals.

In the post-Cairo vision,[12] reproductive health is a major cross-cutting issue, integrating a comprehensive range of services and programmes, including HIV/AIDS and strategies for women's empowerment. Access to good quality, comprehensive, sensitively delivered services, including family planning (there remain significant unmet needs for contraceptive services), are essential to the ability of women and men alike to plan their livelihoods and "invest" adequately in the education and health of their children. Interventions have to be based on an understanding of local customs, traditional beliefs and women's social status. Adolescent reproductive and sexual health must be given higher priority, along with strategies to raise the age of marriage and first childbirth in countries where these remain low. This requires broader interventions in relation to gender empowerment and female education.[13]

Expanding programmes focusing on the priority health needs of the poor

Health interventions should not be limited to these health problems, but programmes focusing on the priority health needs of poor people should be expanded and more effectively targeted to ensure that the poor and socially vulnerable are reached. Combining expanded programmes with more effective targeting (as outlined below) could significantly improve the health of low-income groups and reduce the risk that ill health might lead to poverty. Development agencies should provide support for:

- **The determination of national or local patterns of disease** through epidemiological surveys to facilitate the setting of priorities; an improved understanding of health service utilisation patterns; and the identification of factors inhibiting access to quality health services.

- **Priority setting that takes into account the perspectives of poor people** and is closely linked to actions that address their problems. Finding ways to hear the "voices of the poor", through surveys and through their active participation, is one important way, another is by involving local managers in survey design and analysis and the development and monitoring of the action plans that emerge. Such approaches are essential if programmes are to be well implemented and if communities are to be able to hold health services accountable.

Global Health Initiatives (GHIs) – such as the Expanded Programme on Immunisation and Roll Back Malaria of the WHO, and the Global Alliance for Vaccines and Immunisation (GAVI) – have been initiated in recent years to improve disease control, particularly for poor people. These programmes have reduced disease rates. In addition, some GHIs – such as the GAVI and the Global Fund to Fight AIDS, TB and Malaria (GFATM) – have generated additional resources from the private sector for targeted programmes.[14] But evidence on the longer-term impact of GHIs is less clear. They could make a bigger contribution to better health for poor people if they take a longer-term view, place more emphasis on sustainability, and contribute to the building of national systems. Also, there are issues related to prioritisation, co-ordination and pooled financing that should be addressed.

Box 3. **The role of information and communication technology in pro-poor health systems**

Pro-poor health systems can benefit from an improved and expanded use of ICT in several areas: health education; assisting delivery of care (*e.g.* logistics or diagnosis); knowledge sharing (*e.g.* to keep up with emerging good practice elsewhere); diagnosis (particularly in district and university hospitals); monitoring and statistics for decision making and management – and for keeping track of progress in meeting international targets. This field is ideal for public-private partnership in technology development and capacity development.

Delivering services in difficult partnerships

Some developing countries face more severe constraints to the delivery of effective health interventions than others, though their needs are often even more acute. Some countries with very weak government capacity or those that have recently emerged from conflict have child and maternal mortality rates almost double those in other low-income countries, in part because they have only one third of the number of nurses per capita and double the proportion of the population living in poverty.[15] In such countries, a limited set of interventions or activities may best be delivered in the shorter term through selective use of disease-specific (vertical) programmes.

The advantages of vertical programmes under such circumstances are that they can provide specific technical and financial support targeted against priority diseases such as malaria and tuberculosis that can be more easily controlled and monitored. These programmes can be implemented in partnership with local NGOs, that may have more capacity to deliver general health services and targeted programmes to complement poorly functioning government systems. In conflict countries, "Days of Tranquillity", where fighting is suspended to enable the immunisation of children, have been negotiated during a number of conflicts, and have reportedly had a significant effect on the incidence of diseases such as measles and poliomyelitis.[16] This deserves further evaluation.

The issue of sequencing and the process of capacity building in the health sector are even more crucial in highly constrained environments. Alongside vertical programmes that can address the pressing health needs of poorer populations, measures to strengthen and develop general health service capacity must not be neglected. They require a long-term approach, involving education and training, management strengthening and the development of a sense of ownership in communities and by health workers. An important advantage of strengthening health services in an integrated way is the increased scope for efficiency gains, in economies of scale and scope, as compared to vertical approaches.

3.2. Reaching highly vulnerable groups

In addition to focusing on the poor in general, it is also vital to take special steps to reach the relatively poorest and most vulnerable groups. That requires identifying the most vulnerable groups as well as implementing more effective targeting strategies. As long as services and targeted programmes are of sufficient quality to be attractive to poorer groups they will be utilised (see Section 3.3). Yet although they can be effective, targeting strategies can also be politically sensitive and limited in their coverage. They cannot compensate adequately for the maldistribution of resources common in many partner countries and development agencies, through their dialogue with partner governments, should also urge that budget allocations benefit poor and vulnerable groups.

Identifying vulnerable groups

Identifying the most vulnerable groups may not be possible through income-based definitions of poverty alone, which rarely capture their complexity or gender dimensions. Similarly, it is important to take account of the way that people can move in and out of poverty or become vulnerable to the impoverishing impact of ill health. It is necessary to collect data at regular intervals from household surveys, national indicators, poverty profiles and participatory poverty assessments (PPAs) in order to provide a comprehensive picture.

Data on the health status, health service needs, and the patterns of health service use by vulnerable groups is fundamental to the design of targeting strategies. Experience suggests that the most vulnerable are likely to include the very poor (i.e. the poorest quintile of the population), indigenous people, migrants, adolescents, refugees and socially excluded groups, such as slum-dwellers. Women, particularly the widowed or divorced, are likely to be over-represented, or worse off, in all these groups. These vulnerable groups are often effectively excluded from mainstream services for cultural, administrative and/or geographical reasons. Moreover, there is substantial evidence that highly vulnerable groups are given lower priority by health workers, and thus may be discouraged from attending for care. Training programmes for health workers, which emphasise improving responsiveness, can improve accessibility as long as pay and other incentives for health staff (particularly those working in rural or remote areas) are addressed.[17]

Spatial targeting of vulnerable rural and urban areas

In some countries, remote rural populations have limited access to public health and personal health services. Although poverty is not always geographically concentrated, poverty profiles can be used to facilitate the spatial targeting of vulnerable regions or communities through expanded service coverage, or the allocation of subsidies to non-governmental service providers. There is also evidence that the urban poor can be especially vulnerable and have severely restricted access to urban health services that tend to serve the health needs of the more affluent.[18] Identifying vulnerable urban groups and improving the understanding of their health service needs should also be supported.

Other targeting strategies

Other targeting strategies have been found to be successful under certain circumstances, and merit continuing support from development agencies, with further experimentation and scaling-up as appropriate. For example, the social marketing of commodities such as contraceptives and bed-nets treated with insecticide has been found to benefit primarily middle-income and moderately poor populations; but when complemented by other strategies they have managed to reach more vulnerable populations. The KINET social marketing project in Tanzania, for instance, distributed vouchers through maternal and child health clinics, which was effective in enabling pregnant women to buy treated mosquito nets at a discount.[19]

Targeting refugees

Refugees and the internally displaced are highly vulnerable to disease and ill health. In times of conflict infant mortality typically (but not invariably) increases, the control of preventable diseases (such as measles) is often compromised, and the spread of HIV/AIDS may be exacerbated. The vulnerability of women and young girls substantially rises as economic and social structures weaken, and violence and sexual abuse increase. Mostly as a result of violent conflict, there were an estimated 12 million refugees and 5.3 million internally displaced people in 2001.[20] These people lack access to their usual sources of health care, while the services of host countries or communities become overwhelmed. Getting services – including reproductive health programmes[21] – to these groups is a priority. Humanitarian organisations, primarily local NGOs but also international NGOs and organisations such as the UNHCR and ICRC, are often well placed to deliver services rapidly in such contexts – although care must be taken to work within existing systems and not to undermine them by establishing parallel systems. Consistent with WHO recommendations, development agencies should support the early identification of those most vulnerable, the strengthening of health systems, and the strict co-ordination of activities.

3.3. Increasing demand and participation at community and household levels

Increasing demand for health care

In many countries health service utilisation is low, particularly in the formal public sector. Poor people increasingly turn to private providers for their health care. Understanding of the factors influencing the health-seeking behaviour of poor people is improving though more detailed understanding at the country and district level is necessary for planning purposes.[22] Although cost plays a major role in the decisions of poor people to withdraw from the public sector, there are other important reasons, including:

- **Lack of physical access and inconvenient opening hours** – particularly in sub-Saharan Africa, poor people, especially women, mention long distances to facilities more often than problems of cost or quality.

- **Hidden costs of seeking treatment** – including the opportunity costs of time spent in travel, waiting for treatment, and buying medicines as well as the costs of transport, drugs (supposedly free but often not available) and informal payments demanded by health workers and other staff. These are disincentives to going for treatment, which are aggravated by discrimination in favour of those of higher status and those who could pay bribes.[23]

- **Inadequate or broken equipment and dirty facilities** – a problem exacerbated in many countries by the crisis in public-sector health expenditure and routine underfunding of primary services and of non-salary recurrent costs.

- **Absenteeism and lack of staff** – doctors and other health workers are often absent from their posts, sometimes because their salaries are inadequate or may not have been paid for several months, requiring them to seek other income-generating opportunities during working hours.

- **The behaviour of medical and health staff** – rude, disrespectful treatment of poor people is widespread and almost universally complained about; public-sector facilities are often singled out as particularly bad. In Ethiopia, for example, government health centres and hospitals score badly on staff attitude and behaviour; the staff of NGO and mission facilities are more frequently cited as providing better treatment.[24] Many studies of low utilisation of formal health services by poor women have emphasised the importance of respectful and sensitive treatment by providers.

- **Quality of services and availability of drugs** – for the poor, all of these problems combine into a general complaint about quality of care. In Borg Meghezel, Egypt, for instance, people received what is meant to be free medical care but villagers reported that the clinic had no drugs and that the doctor had turned it into his private clinic.[25]

For these and other reasons – such as lack of education and understanding of health problems, or lower priority being given to the health needs of women and girls – the take-up rate of health services is often low. So steps have to be taken to address these issues. The main objective is to provide visibly effective quality interventions, which will itself stimulate demand and lead to increased utilisation. In the longer run, the education of poor people, particularly of women, will help them to seek out health services and to campaign for improvements in coverage and quality.

Promoting community participation

- **More widespread use of strategies that improve the availability and use of information in the community are recommended.** Demand is constrained by a lack of understanding about what is good and what is bad for health, as well as poor knowledge of where to find preventive and curative interventions. Strategies would include: targeted information campaigns with the active participation of communities; improving access to information on the performance of providers and on the purchasing of health goods and services; and helping poor people to make choices about health services. This help could come, for example, through the mandatory and clear posting of prices at facilities; the dissemination of simple and clear information on the quality of local providers; and information campaigns on safe use of over-the-counter drugs and on distinguishing counterfeit or out-of-date supplies.

- **Programmes that increase the numbers of health workers and "facilitators" working in communities can be an effective vehicle for bringing more information on health promotion and services to households.**[26] In turn, such programmes can channel information on the needs and demands of communities, especially the most vulnerable groups, back to local health services. The state of Andhra Pradesh in India has recorded some notable successes in using facilitators, usually women chosen by the community, in poor urban areas to raise awareness and act as a bridge between communities and facilities. Further experimentation and expansion with such programmes should be supported by development agencies.

- **More emphasis should be placed, too, on meaningful community participation,** while recognising that communities are not homogeneous entities.[27] Although the health sector has for many years been an area for pilot approaches in civil society participation, poor people and communities typically have little voice in decisions about health service provision despite the desirability of their being able to express their rights and influence the state institutions and social processes that affect their lives. In some countries, civil society has been too weak to address failures of government health provision, and health reforms have been decided without sufficient consultation with local stakeholders.

- **It is critical that the voices of the poor, particularly women, are given due attention** both in the targeting of resources, and in the design, content and financing of pro-poor health services. Evidence shows that community participation and ownership of health services can contribute to increased use, improved patient satisfaction and knowledge, and strengthened community capacities.

- **Interest has also turned to the potential of civil society groups to improve the accountability of health services, both public and private.** The active involvement of communities can be an effective tool for improving performance and strengthening links with health services in remote districts and can contribute to an overall improvement in governance, provided this involvement is not captured by elites to the detriment of poorer people – and particularly women. Involving communities and civil society organisations also has the potential to increase advocacy on behalf of poor people, who do not have easy or regular – if, indeed, any – access to legal or other formal means of redress. In Zimbabwe, for example, a strong alliance of civil society stakeholders from trade unions, NGOs and informal associations has been involved in monitoring policies and expenditures across the health sector.[28]

● **The PRS process must be informed by improved consultation** within the health sector, as a part of a broader approach to participation. In addition, improved education, particularly of women, will both increase appropriate use and enable communities to voice their needs to national and local governments.

4. Provider pluralism and the challenge of health service delivery

Health service delivery has become increasingly diverse. In many countries, not least in sub-Saharan Africa and in the poorer parts of Asia, the private sector (see Box 4) is a major provider of health services. In many countries, too, particularly in some transitional countries such as China and parts of the Newly Independent States of the former Soviet Union, public health workers and facilities are in effect selling their services and acting as *de facto* private providers. Users are thus faced with an increasingly pluralistic set-up that offers many types of provider. They are generally described under the broad term "private sector", but it is important to be very clear as to the heterogeneity of "private" provision and thus of the policy and strategic challenges that it raises.

4.1. Use of private sector services

Use of both private for-profit and not-for-profit services by the poor is variable, both across and within countries. There are examples of extensive use by poor people.[29] High rates of use are found in some countries for reproductive and child health services.[30] In other countries, though, the public sector is the main provider of preventive and basic health services, with recourse to private services for curative care for adults. Use of private services may substitute for, or coexist with, the use of public-sector services by the poor.[31] In some countries poor women and girls are particularly likely to seek access to private services because they are more convenient or more readily accessible, or are more respectful in their treatment. It may be easier for women to visit such providers without a male escort, or there may be a gender bias towards treatment for men and boys from professional providers, and treatment of girls and women by unqualified or traditional practitioners. In all countries, the purchase of drugs from local or itinerant drug-sellers is a common first-line strategy for the poor, though few data are available on which types of private provision the poor use the most, and in what order of preference.

Reasons for the growth in private provision will vary according to context, but they are largely related to the problems of public provision identified in Section 3.3. In countries such as China, where there has been a radical change in the nature of public services and rapid development of private-for-profit markets, there has been a widespread increase in self-treatment across all socio-economic groups. As a result, commercial pharmacies, shopkeepers and local drug-sellers now account for substantial amounts of household expenditure on health.

As noted above, the relationship between the public and private sectors is not straightforward and what is public and what is private is increasingly porous. Public-sector health staff frequently work privately, charging fees for services, often unregistered and unsupervised. Public-sector facilities are often chronically under funded and in many countries staff have to market their skills and services in order to make a living. Uganda is one such country.[32] And since fiscal decentralisation in China, only about 15% of health workers' salaries are met by government funds; the remainder has to be made up by sales of drugs and services.[33] Indeed, the public sector in some countries resembles a private-for-profit sector with a public subsidy.

Box 4. **What is the private health sector?**

There are differing views on the definition of the private sector. For some it is limited to for-profit activities. For others it is a diversity of health service providers working outside the formal government sector, whether their aim is commercial or philanthropic. Here the latter, broader, definition is used. The private sector includes both registered and unregistered providers operating under a diversity of organisational and contractual arrangements:

● Not-for-profit providers include NGOs and faith-based organisations, which operate primary health care clinics and secondary level hospitals. Many of these organisations bring services to rural and under-served areas and receive external finance, operating (for example) under a contract or agreement with the government.

● A range of non-profit-making community-based organisations, civil society groups, voluntary support groups, and other charitable institutions also provide health and support services. They may be formal or informal and may also be involved in awareness-raising activities, counselling and home-based care. The HIV/AIDS epidemic has led to the development of many small, informal groups, which provide invaluable support to people living with HIV/AIDS.

● The for-profit sector includes qualified health and allied practitioners working individually or for profit-based institutions such as clinics, hospitals, pharmacies and laboratories. They generally operate under licence, although enforcement may be lax. A large proportion of these private practitioners may also work for the government. Unlicensed pharmacists and drug-peddlers provide the first line of health services in many countries. They often number in the thousands, operate from home or small market-stalls and provide a range of medical goods such as drugs (both restricted and unrestricted) and contraceptives.

● Finally, there are many community-based traditional practitioners such as birth attendants and healers from various indigenous medical systems. They may charge a fee, take payment in kind or offer services on a reciprocal basis. They are mostly unregulated by governments but some countries have set up registered practitioner associations.

In countries where there are moderate problems of governance and where the public health sector has come under increasing strain, high degrees of pluralism in the provision of health services often exist with few or no checks on the competence of the provider.[34] As a result, the private sector is often extremely diverse in its capacity to deliver appropriate, competent services. This plurality has the advantage of allowing both profit- and non-profit-making providers to provide the services that the public sector cannot, thus extending coverage to poor and non-poor alike. On the other hand, in such difficult situations, the poor often do not have the funds to afford those services available in the profit-making sector that are of high quality, or access services in the non-profit sector which are limited by funding in their availability.

4.2. Developing partnerships with the private sector

Governments should engage more proactively with the private sector to ensure that it is contributing to the achievement of pro-poor health objectives. The type of relationship that can be developed will depend on a contextual analysis of existing patterns of use, the relative strength and quality of different kinds of providers, and the capacity of government to develop and implement effective regulatory, contracting and other mechanisms. A wide range of approaches has been used to date,[35] including co-operation with informal-sector practitioners and offering training and supplies, the contracting of diagnostic tasks (*e.g.* laboratory and imaging services) to private organisations, and contracting out service provision. Some of these strategies can provide useful models for replication by governments and development agencies in other countries so long as the impact on the health status of vulnerable groups is properly evaluated. For example:

- **The provision of public subsidies to non-government providers** as a mechanism for improving the quality of, and access to, services in under-served locations. Contracting out of provision for specific services or for entire districts has been done on a pilot basis in Cambodia. A pilot programme evaluating different models of service contracting to NGOs found that service utilisation increased by the largest amount where NGOs were given the entire responsibility for hiring and managing staff.[36] In sub-Saharan Africa agreements have been made with church organisations that provide the mainstay of service delivery in some areas. In other countries NGOs perform the same function; BEMFAM in Brazil, for example, is a major supplier of high-quality reproductive health services in poor rural and urban localities. Specification of the quantity and quality of services has to be built into such agreements, service delivery monitored, and capacity built in areas of national priority. Development agencies can facilitate this type of public-private partnership by helping strengthen capacity in contracting and monitoring.

- **Working with informal and commercial providers** as in the training of traditional birth attendants and other informal practitioners, have been supported by development co-operation agencies; the results have been mixed. More recently, the HIV/AIDS epidemic has led to some innovative programmes, such as the training of unlicensed pharmacists as peer health educators (because of their extensive contacts with youth and men), and supplying pre-packaged STD drugs to retail outlets. Traditional healers also assume important functions in home care for people living with HIV/AIDS in highly affected African countries.[37] Training has improved the skill of private providers in India in diagnosing and treating TB and has helped shopkeepers in Kenya provide the correct anti-malarial drugs. Development agencies should consider ongoing experimentation in this area with support for the analysis of impact on the health status of poor and vulnerable groups.

- **Developing regulatory frameworks.** These exist in most countries in some format (except where they have collapsed, as in failed or weak states, or where they are being renegotiated because of transition, such as in China). But enforcement tends to be lax. The Consumer Protection Act in India (COPRA) is one attempt to create a legal framework of redress. Although it has had limited impact, cases can now be brought against private medical practitioners under COPRA. Chances of success are low (around 30%) and access is *de facto* limited to higher-income groups, but information flows to consumers have improved as a consequence.[38] Frameworks are also not necessarily appropriate for changing situations. In Thailand, for example, in the context of an economic boom, a policy of encouraging private-sector expansion of hospitals without an adequate regulatory environment had adverse consequences for the public health sector, including a brain drain towards the private sector and the accumulation of high-cost medical technology that was under used.[39] To ensure that private-sector initiatives contribute to public health objectives a variety of mechanisms, involving a range of different stakeholders, can be used to enable more effective checks and balances to emerge without suppressing private-sector initiatives. Development agencies can facilitate the sharing of lessons on private-sector management across countries while helping build capacity in regulation.

● **Other strategies** for working with the private sector that have been effective include: social marketing programmes that expand demand for and supply of primary commodities such as contraceptives; working with civil society to improve the accountability of health services; and improving the availability of information on provider performance as described in Section 3.3.

4.3. Output-based approaches to aid

One approach to contractual arrangements – an output-based approach to aid (OBA) – is being tested by the World Bank (see Box 5).

Box 5. **Output-based approaches to aid**

There is increasing discussion of the possibility of using output-based approaches to aid (OBA) in the health sector, whereby development agencies or governments delegate the delivery of services to the private sector (for-profit and not-for-profit alike) on the basis of the achievement of specific outputs. OBAs are one of several means by which governments can finance the provision of services by non-government providers and should not be confused with the more traditional approach of financing or subsidising the estimated cost of inputs. Development agencies have been supporting this more traditional approach for some time and it has proven effective in many cases in delivering support for the poor in under-served areas and in adverse conditions. The objective of OBA is to increase incentives for efficiency, to enhance accountability in the use of public resources, and to create opportunities to mobilise private financing. Proponents argue that the likelihood of implementation is increased through payment by results, and benefits from market competition. There is little consensus, though, about the extent to which output-based delivery of health services is appropriate, and for which type of services. There are also issues similar to those now under debate in OECD countries of the advantages and disadvantages of financing on the basis of "capitation". In cases of weak governance, there would be more opportunities for cutting corners and for fraud. It is likely to be most readily applicable where outputs can be easily defined and their relationship with health outcomes is clear (immunisation is an example). Where applied, OBAs should be integrated into the overall health programme.

---

5. Developing equitable health financing mechanisms

5.1. Health financing and social protection

The objective of health financing should be to assure the availability of funding, as well as to set the right incentives for providers, and to ensure that all individuals have access to effective public health and personal health care. Existing resources allocated to health in developing countries are inadequate to finance a health system that meets the needs of poor people. Some increases in government spending for health are possible through budget reallocations, efficiency savings, and the use of funds released from debt relief. Yet the poorest countries will remain unable to provide sufficient resources to meet pro-poor health objectives without a substantial increase in external financing.

- **Health financing systems have important consequences for the degree of protection against ill health.** An equitable financing strategy should ensure financial protection for everyone and eliminate the possibility of poor people being unable to pay for their health care, or becoming impoverished as a result. The design and implementation of health financing mechanisms is the responsibility of several government departments beyond the ministry of health, such as ministries of finance and social welfare, and social security departments. Dialogue between all the main actors, including development agencies, on protecting access for poor people is essential.

- **The ways in which health systems are financed also have important gender dimensions.** Women have less access to personal income (limiting their ability to pay user fees or insurance contributions) and a lower share of household expenditure for their health needs. In addition, they are disadvantaged by biases in insurance and other pre-payment schemes (*e.g.* computation of actuarial risk, exclusion of maternity conditions), whereas their needs – particularly for reproductive health services – are high.

- **Issues of health system financing are closely related to broader issues of social protection,** which include considerations of macro-economic stability in national economies. Health-specific protection measures should be designed and implemented in conjunction with other approaches to provide basic protection against the "shocks" likely to lead to poverty and in turn worsen health status.[40] The poor and socially vulnerable are exposed to multiple risks from different sources, which require different forms of risk management instruments and strategies for given populations (in families and communities or through NGOs, market institutions or government agencies).[41] In particular, poor households are obliged to prioritise expenditure of finite income; the amount of out-of-pocket spending available for health care will depend on the amounts spent on other strategic social costs, such as education, as well as on amounts needed for basic subsistence.

- **Health services – public or private – are financed by a number of different mechanisms.** In view of the low public expenditures on health in many partner countries, out-of-pocket expenditures (user fees) can account for 20 to 80% of health expenditures.[42] Evidence shows that requiring payment at the time of illness restricts access to health services by the poor, and may deny basic care to the poorest members of society. Even middle-income households are vulnerable to impoverishment if a member has a catastrophic illness requiring costly health care, or if sickness means that an income-earner cannot work.

5.2. Risk-sharing and pre-payment approaches

Pooling is the accumulation and management of revenues to ensure that the risk of having to pay for health care is borne by all members of the pool. It is traditionally known as the "insurance function", whether explicit (people subscribe to an insurance scheme) or implicit (through tax revenues). Pre-payment and risk-pooling predominate in developed countries where revenue is collected by general taxation or social insurance and the pool is large, but it is rare in low-income countries – and for partner countries the development of large pools with cross-subsidisation, or well-regulated multiple pools, would be an important step forward. Health financing policy should therefore focus on creating the conditions for the development of the largest possible pooling arrangements.[43]

The feasibility of pooling and risk-sharing depends on the country involved. In the many low-income countries without the organisational, financial or institutional capacity to create a large pool, policy makers, with development agency support, should try and create the conditions in which they can arise. Even relatively small pools are preferable to pure out-of-pocket payment. Agencies can support the development of employment-based contribution schemes and community or provider-based pre-payment schemes as a transition to larger pools or more targeted subsidies. Some countries (China is one) are experimenting with medical safety nets for rural households in designated poor areas to cover the costs of major illnesses, particularly hospital admissions by the very poor.

Community schemes – those managed by community groups or NGOs, and serving people in a defined locality – must aim to build and draw on community solidarity by, for example, ensuring widespread enrolment and mechanisms for control by the community. In some cases, it may be possible to include health insurance in the programmes of broader community-based organisations, such as income-generating schemes. One advantage is that these organisations are likely to have stronger management capacity. Micro-insurance schemes – voluntary insurance schemes with most participants at or below the poverty line – are becoming more widespread and are providing experience that can be built upon.[44] Community schemes have demonstrated some small-scale success, but more evaluation and efforts at larger-scale replication are required.

In the poorest countries, where risk-pooling cannot generate adequate social protection, health-sector budgets – supplemented by external assistance or debt relief channelled to the health sector – must play a role for the foreseeable future. This approach assumes that such additional resources will be allocated in a pro-poor fashion. In middle-income countries, tax-based health financing could be expanded. Alternatively, access could be improved by strengthening and expanding existing mandatory employment-based health insurance schemes to include more informal workers and subsidise their participation.

5.3. Cost-sharing approaches and user fees

In many partner countries, resource constraints and concerns about the inefficiencies of public-sector services have led to reforms in health financing prioritising revenue generation and efficiency objectives over equity concerns. This approach has led to the introduction of, or an increase in, user fees. As poverty reduction becomes central to government policy, ministries of health and finance are increasingly concerned with the ways that user fees affect the poor.

The evidence of the impact of user fees in the public sector largely demonstrates that they reduce the take-up of services by the poor and that exemption systems have failed to identify and protect the poor from their impact.[45] The use of primary services by the poor is already influenced by time and opportunity costs and user fees tend to *ration* further use. The abolition of user fees in Uganda as part of the poverty-reduction strategy resulted in a surge of utilisation by the poor, though in South Africa, by contrast, the withdrawal of user fees for maternal and child health services did not lead to a substantial increase in use.[46] But, given that government expenditures are currently too low to finance essential health services, and that private expenditures represent over half of health spending in many countries, user fees remain an important aspect of health financing policy in most low-income countries. And user fees (in the form of co-payments) also are the general rule, to varying extents, in OECD countries. Indeed in some partner countries, budget constraints and political pressure have led to the reinstatement of previously withdrawn user fees.[47]

User fees therefore have to be approached cautiously in order to ensure that the access of poor people to quality health services is protected. With strong attention to this issue, a combination of approaches according to national circumstances may be appropriate. Subject to fiscal limits, these may include:

- **Free primary-level services.** Accessing primary health care services is extremely important to poor people. User fees for primary care have rarely been effective in generating sufficient amounts of resources to lead to sustained improvements in the quality of services. As discussed above, encouraging free provision of primary services will increase access.

- **Free services for targeted groups or communities.** The identification of highly vulnerable groups and communities has been discussed in Section 3. Targeting groups such as indigenous people, adolescents or refugees with free services can be highly effective in increasing access. The same point applies to identifying very poor communities or districts for free provision of services.

- **Free services for priority diseases and conditions.** Some health conditions are responsible for a considerable proportion of the burden of ill health borne by the poor. Diagnosis and treatment of these conditions could be exempt from charges, regardless of the health facility where services are received. For example, exempting health care for children, obstetric and reproductive health care, and the management of STDs and TB would have a considerable impact on the health outcomes of the poor. Criteria for exemptions would have to be determined according to local patterns of diseases and the priority requirements of poor groups. This strategy has been used in Ghana, leading to increased coverage of the exempted interventions, although the budget allocation for exemptions was inadequate.[48]

- **Exemption systems for hospital services (district or secondary level).** The high costs of hospitalisation, even in district hospitals, can be a major source of impoverishment. The need for exemption systems targeted on vulnerable groups, but including those above the poverty line that may be forced into poverty as a result of hospital charges, is critical. Countries such as Uganda and Bangladesh are experimenting with hospital-based exemption systems or the cross-subsidisation of poorer patients by private patients.

- **Charges for the use of university or highly specialised hospital services by those who can afford to pay,** and who tend to get highly disproportionate use of these services, should not be subsidised with public funds. There will, of course, be political resistance to eliminating or sharply reducing these subsidies to the better off. When people on low incomes are referred through the health care system to such facilities, some system of exemption from charges is clearly desirable.

Some countries are trying to develop objective and non-stigmatising exemption systems in order to allow some degree of cost-recovery while maintaining access for poor people. In the NGO sector, community involvement and monitoring, plus community setting of fees, have made user fees more successful in balancing equity and efficiency (see Box 6). Development agencies can support more innovative approaches to cost-recovery and social insurance, while improving in the analysis of the social impact, so that any adverse effects on poor people, and on women in particular, can be identified early.[49]

Box 6. **The Aga Khan Health Service approach to user fees**

The Aga Khan Health Services (AKHS) in Pakistan has an extensive network of primary health centres and first-level referral facilities in the Northern Areas and Chitral District. These services are designed to meet the health care needs of women and children in remote villages principally reliant on subsistence agriculture. Services have been planned in close consultation with communities which provide in-kind support for the construction of the centres and who nominate persons to be trained as community health workers by AKHS. Clients pay a fee for most services, although the fees vary between communities and are negotiated with each community. In negotiating the fee, community leadership seeks to achieve a balance between a fee which is generally affordable in that particular village and a fee which covers an increasing percentage of the direct operating cost of providing the service. Some of the more prosperous villages have set fees at rates that have enabled the community to cover direct operating costs within five years. For most villages, however, it is mutually agreed between the village leadership and AKHS that 10 to 15 years will be necessary before this degree of cost recovery can be achieved. In the interim, AKHS subsidises the service.

Experience to date indicates that this approach covers most members of a given community but does not adequately ensure access to the poorest households in some villages. To reach the very poor, a welfare policy has to be put in place by the village leadership, supported by AKHS. The current welfare approach consists of exemptions for particularly disadvantaged families. But it is threatened by downturns in regional economic performance and the seasonality of incomes. Additional approaches to welfare, including per capita contributions from the ministry of health for the very poor, are being explored.

Strategies to reduce the direct financial burden of health care must also tackle the unofficial fees imposed by health-sector staff which are often higher than official user fees, are demanded by allied staff (such as cleaners) and health professionals, and are a major deterrent to take-up. The publication and posting of official charges, more community involvement in health facility management, and improved governance will all contribute. In addition, addressing the incentives of health-sector staff is important.

Notes

1. In Mali, for instance, communities were successfully given the right to hire health workers on their own and to negotiate conditions, which at the same time reinforced the accountability of health workers to the local population.

2. Improving information and communication networks (through ICT) can create powerful social and economic networks and have a role to play in improving health systems. See Action Point 7 – ICT for health care, G8's Genoa Plan of Action.

3. For example, Ghana successfully decentralised health service management through strengthening district management systems and restructuring the Ministry of Health. The creation of a strong cadre of public health doctor/managers at all tiers of the system was an important element in this process, as were long-term external funding and technical advice.

4. Murray, C.J.L. and A.D. Lopez (eds.) (1996), *Global Health Statistics* (Global Burden of Disease and Injury Series, Volume II), Cambridge, Massachusetts.

5. Prabhat, J. and F. Chaloupka (1999), *Curbing the Epidemic: Governments and the Economics of Tobacco Control*, World Bank, Washington.

6. Maternal mortality is generally defined as death during pregnancy or within 42 days of termination of pregnancy from any cause related to, or aggravated by, the pregnancy or its management.

7. UNICEF (1996), *The Progress of Nations*, UNICEF, New York.

8. Alan Guttmacher Institute (1999), "Abortion in Context: United States and Worldwide", *Issues in Brief*, Series No. 1, Alan Guttmacher Institute, USA.

9. Safe Motherhood Inter-Agency Group, "Implementing the Safe Motherhood Action Agenda: A resource guide" *Safe Motherhood Resource Guide* Accessible at *www.safemotherhood.org/smrg/overview/overview.htm* .

10. Ashford, L. (2002), "Hidden Suffering: Disabilities From Pregnancy and Childbirth in Less Developed Countries", *Health Reports*, Population Reference Bureau.

11. Safe Motherhood Inter-Agency Group, *op. cit.*

12. The International Conference on Population and Development held in Cairo in 1994.

13. UNFPA (United Nations Population Fund) (1999), "Six Billion: a time for choices", (Chapter 3, Reproductive Health and Reproductive Rights), *State of the World Population 1999*, UNFPA, New York.

14. The GFATM has received pledges of approximately USD 2.2 billion, of which just under 5 % has been pledged by private donors.

15. WHO (2002), *Improving Health Outcomes of the Poor*, Report of Working Group 5 of the Commission on Macroeconomics and Health, WHO, Geneva.

16. WHO (2002), *World Report on Violence and Health*, WHO, Geneva.

17. Vlassof, C. (2001), "Health Workers for Change, A Quality of Care Intervention", *Health Policy and Planning*, No. 16 (Supplement No. 1).

18. Werna, E. (2001), *Combating Urban Inequalities Challenges for Managing Cities in the Developing World*, Edward Elgar, Aldershot, UK.

19. Schellenberg J. R. *et al.* (2001), "Effect of large-scale social marketing of insecticide-treated nets on child survival in rural Tanzania", *Lancet* 357: 1241-1247.

20. UNHCR (United Nations High Commission For Refugees) (2002), *Refugees by Numbers*, Accessible at *www.unhcr.ch*

21. UNFPA (2002), *The Impact of Conflict on Women and Girls: Strategy for Gender Mainstreaming in Areas of Conflict and Reconstruction.* Accessible at www.unfpa.org/publications/armedconflict_women.pdf UNFPA (undated) *Reproductive Health for Communities in Crisis: UNFPA Emergency Response.* Accessible at *www.unfpa.org/modules/intercenter/crisis/crisis_eng.pdf*

22. Narayan, D. *et al.* (2000), *Voices of the Poor Crying out for Change*, World Bank, Washington. See also Milimo, J., T. Shilito and K. Brock (2002), "The poor of Zambia speak: Who would ever listen to the poor?", *Findings from Participatory Research on Poverty in Zambia in the 1990s*, Zambia Social Investment Fund.

23. *Ibid.* pp. 101–2.

24. Tolossa, A. and R. Lambert (1997), *Participatory Rural Assessment of Community Perceptions of Quality of Health Care Services in East Haraghe, Ethiopia*, Save the Children Fund, London.

25. Narayan, D. (2000), *op. cit.* pp. 103–4.

26. Kahssay, H.M., M.E. Taylor and P.A. Berman (1998), Community Health Workers: The Way Forward, *Public Health in Action* No. 4, WHO, Geneva.

27. Oakley, P. (1989), *Community Involvement in Health Development: An Examination of the Critical Issues*, WHO, Geneva; and Kahssay, H.M. and P. Oakley (eds.) (1999), *Community Involvement in Health Development. A review of the concept and practice*, WHO, Geneva.

28. Loewenson, R. (1999), "Public Participation in Health: making people matter", *IDS Working Paper No. 84*, Institute of Development Studies and Training and Research Support Centre (TARSC).

29. For example, a survey of private-sector clinic patients in Ghana found 50% were from the low-income group; a household survey in Rajasthan in India found that 80% of the users of private-sector childcare were in the poorer-income groups. See Sharma, S. (2001), *The Private Sector and Child Health Care*, Carolina Consulting Corporation, Chapel Hill, NC. Accessible at *www.futuresgroup.com/documents/final_-_WHO_2.pdf*

30. See *ibid.* on utilisation for child care. For reproductive health, see Rannan-Eliya, R.P. *et al.* (2000), *Expenditures for Reproductive Health and Family Planning Services in Egypt and Sri Lanka.* Accessible at *www.policyproject.com/pubs/commissionedresearch/harvard.pdf*

31. Sharma, S. (2001), *op. cit.*

32. McPake, B. *et al.* (1999), "Informal Economic Activities of Public Health Workers in Uganda: Implications for Quality and Accessibility", *Social Science and Medicine* Vol. 49, No. 7: pp. 849–65.

33. Bloom, G. and X. Gu (1997), "Health Sector Reform: lessons from China", *Social Science and Medicine*, Vol. 45, No. 3: pp. 351-360.

34. Bloom, G. and H. Standing (2001), "Pluralism and Marketisation in the Health Sector", *IDS Working Paper No. 136,* Institute of Development Studies, University of Sussex.

35. Mills, A. *et al.* (2002), "What can be done about the private health sector in low-income countries?", *Bulletin of the World Health Organization,* Vol. 80, No. 4: pp. 325–30. See also Smith, E. *et al.* (2001), *Working with Private Sector Providers for Better Health Care: An Introductory Guide,* Options/London School of Hygiene and Tropical Medicine, London.

36. Loevinsohn, B. (2000), *Contracting for the Delivery of Primary Health Care in Cambodia: design and experience of a large pilot project.* Accessible at www.worldbank.org/wbi/health/flagship/oj_cambodia.pdf

37. UNAIDS (2001), *Reaching Out and Scaling Up: Eight Case Studies of Home and Community Care for and by People with HIV/AIDS.* Accessible at *www.unaids.org/publications/documents/persons/JC608-ReachOut-E.pdf*

38. Bhat, R. (1996), "Regulating the Private Health Care Sector: The Case of the Indian Consumer Protection Act", *Health Policy and Planning* Vol. 11, No. 3: 266-279.

39. Bennett, S. and V. Tangcharoensathien (1994), "A Shrinking State? Politics, Economics and Private Health are in Thailand", *Public Administration and Development,* Vol. 14, No. 1: pp. 1–17.

40. Such "shocks" include loss of income because of unemployment, loss of assets (from natural disasters, for example), as well as disability and lack of support in old age through the loosening of family and kinship structures.

41. World Bank (2002), *Social Protection Sector Strategy: From Safety Net to Springboard,* World Bank, Washington.

42. WHO (2000), *The World Health Report 2000 - Health Systems: Improving Performance,* WHO, Geneva.

43. *Ibid.*

44. ILO (International Labour Organization) (2000), *Health Micro-insurance: A Compendium,* Working Paper. Accessible at www.gdrc.org/icm/step-ilo.html

45. Gilson, L. (1997), "The Lessons of User Fees Experience in Africa", *Health Policy and Planning,* Vol. 12, No. 4: pp. 273–85.

46. Schneider, H. and L. Gilson (1999), "The impact of free maternal health care in South Africa". IN Berer, M. and T.K. Sundari Ravindran (eds), *Safe motherhood initiatives: critical issues,* Reproductive Health Matters, Blackwell Science, Oxford, UK.

47. Foster, M. and S. Mackintosh-Walker (2001), *Sector-Wide Programmes and Poverty Reduction,* Overseas Development Institute, London.

48. *Ibid.*

49. This is already a requirement of PRGF-supported programmes.

ISBN 92-64-10018-0
DAC Guidelines and Reference Documents
Poverty and Health
© OECD, WHO 2003

Chapter 3

Key Policy Areas for Pro-poor Health

Abstract.   Ensuring that the poor have access to effective and affordable health services is central to a pro-poor health approach. However, it is not sufficient in itself to improve the health of the poor since major determinants of their health depend on actions beyond the health sector. There is, indeed, ample and long-standing evidence of the effects of a range of sectoral policies and macro-economic practices on health outcomes. Those that are critically important include education, food security, safe water, sanitation and energy. The health of the poor can also be improved by reducing their exposure to air pollution, violence, injuries at home, in the workplace, and on the roads, and by preventing the devastating impact of conflict and natural disasters. Development agencies can support policies in these sectors that promote health and poverty reduction objectives.

1. Introduction

The contribution of sectoral policies to heath objectives may be beneficial or adverse and the impact increased through interactive effects between them. Consequently, it is important to prioritise those sectors that have a major impact on health and poverty reduction, and assess the extent to which policies promote or undermine both health and broader poverty reduction objectives. This prioritisation points to the importance of strengthening capacity within these sectors for the attainment of health objectives. The following sections highlight linkages between poverty, health and other important sectors. Some of them, as with health and education, are well known. Others like interpersonal violence and road traffic injuries are less obvious but important as causes of death and ill-health. Recommendations for development agencies, in support of the achievement of health objectives through action in these sectors, are then outlined.

Figure 2. **The Main Determinants of Health**

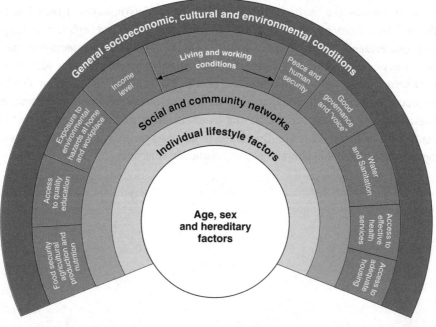

Adapted from: Dahlgren, G. and M. Whitehead (1991), *Policies and Strategies to Promote Social Equity in Health*, Institute of Futures Studies, Stockholm.

2. Education as a tool for improved health outcomes

Education and health are fundamental to poverty reduction and feature directly in five of the eight MDGs. Achievement of the three health-related goals hinges strongly on reaching the goals of universal primary education and the closely related goal of gender

DAC GUIDELINES AND REFERENCE SERIES: POVERTY AND HEALTH – ISBN 92-64-10018-0 – © OECD, WHO 2003

equality. *The evidence demonstrating inter-linkages between investments in health and education and their synergetic effects on reducing poverty is compelling.* Yet in many partner countries a lack of appropriate investment has left the education sector in weak condition. Inadequate infrastructure, a lack of learning materials, poorly trained and demotivated teachers with no access to continuing education programmes, overburdened curricula, and over-centralised decision-making have all contributed to a general failure in meeting education targets. Those low-income countries that have given priority to investments in education have nonetheless lowered mortality levels far below those countries with much higher per capita incomes but less well educated populations.

Minds and bodies – education and health – are the most important assets of poor people, enabling them to lead socially and economically productive lives. Even a few years of schooling provide basic skills that can have far-reaching implications for health-seeking behaviour. Moreover, education emphasising health prevention and informed self-help is among the most effective ways of empowering the poor to take charge of their own lives.

Key linkages with poverty and health

Findings from numerous studies have clarified the nature of the link between education and health, showing that:

- **Female education is strongly related to improved health care for children, families, and communities.** One of the most powerful means to reduced child mortality is the literacy of mothers, itself the product of an education system that ensures access to education for the poor, girls as well as boys. Stronger receptivity and confidence – just as much as the knowledge acquired in school – enable women to apply the advice given by health personnel. Beyond its effect on personal behaviour, the literacy of mothers is critical for all kinds of health interventions, including increasing the access of family members and the broader community to the formal health care system.[1]

- **Education is related to lower fertility rates.** Education leads to changes in reproductive behaviour which produce a series of beneficial effects: lower maternal mortality, female empowerment, higher survival rates for children, spacing of births, improved health of mothers and children, better care for children, lower desired and achieved fertility rates, and reduced poverty.

- **Education is one of the most effective tools against HIV/AIDS.** Since learning at an early age is critical in shaping future behaviour, young people are both especially vulnerable and open to change. This holds true for health, too, where more than two-thirds of premature adult deaths can be ascribed to behavioural patterns acquired in adolescence. Information, education and communication campaigns,[2] peer education, youth centres and community-based services may play a crucial role, especially in the case of sexual and reproductive health.

Exploiting the synergies between health and education

Although education is essential for health improvement, *health is also a major determinant of educational attainment:* it has a direct impact on cognitive abilities and school attendance. Policy makers and staff in the two sectors therefore have a mutual interest in interacting closely and identifying strategies for collaboration using both the school system and informal education channels.

The role of formal education in promoting health. Many developing country governments recognise the potential of schools and other education centres for fulfilling multiple health functions. Development agencies can support the efforts of partner countries to strengthen the use of schools for health promotion by stepping up technical and financial assistance for the three key functions of school health programmes.

- **The main elements of school-based health services** are immunisation, health monitoring and referral, nutritional supplements, and feeding programmes. Schools can provide an important focus for improving nutrition. A well-functioning school health programme is one of the most cost-effective ways of preventing ill health. But the current state of both health and education systems in many low-income countries means that programmes are often non-functional. Additional resources are required, together with system reform, training, and close collaboration between the health and education sectors, both among ministries and schools themselves.

- **Health education in school provides scope for joint initiatives and training by health workers and teachers.** Different approaches may be used to integrate health education into school curricula: integrating health education into science and other relevant topics, for example, or teaching it as a stand-alone subject with compulsory student examination. Whichever method is used, it is important that health education as a subject is not marginalised by teachers or students. Teachers are in a position to transfer health knowledge and promote healthy behaviour. But in countries where school children, particularly girls, have been shown to be vulnerable to sexual exploitation by teachers, inputs by health professionals may be necessary. For their part, health professionals have a key role in designing appropriate school curricula and in training teachers.

- **The school also has a role in community health**, particularly in rural areas, where it can be a means of introducing behavioural change and basic health concepts in the children's home. Education and health are both sectors that can motivate parental involvement and, by acting in synergy through school health programmes, can generate effective community participation and well-being, and can also help empower communities.

The role of non-formal education in promoting health. Since many poor people, especially girls and women, do not have access to formal education, it is important to focus also on those outside the formal school system. Efforts to promote health must reach out to vulnerable young people, such as street children, sex workers and the million of orphans whose parents have died of AIDS or in violent conflict. Integrating health education into non-formal education and functional literacy programmes offers the potential to reach at least some within these vulnerable groups. In addition, the use of the mass media and peer education deserves special attention.

Recommendations to development agencies

To develop the potential of education for protecting and improving the health of the poor, development agencies should capitalise on the synergies between health and education by supporting partner countries in:

- **Promoting the achievement of the education-related MDGs** since primary education and female literacy are decisive factors influencing the health of the most vulnerable and poorest groups of population.

- **Tackling barriers to female education** in schools, such as the personal safety of girls when they are travelling to school and also inside schools, or enabling pregnant girls to continue their schooling.

● **Strengthening the use of schools for health promotion** by stepping up technical and financial assistance for school health programmes, which requires joint actions by education and health personnel to strengthen the school as a focal point for health education and health-service delivery. This co-operation should include teacher training, the introduction of health topics in school curricula, the provision of school meals and the strengthening of school health services.

● **Integrating health training into non-formal education** and functional literacy programmes, including assisting the development of an enabling environment for NGOs to carry out health education in non-formal settings.

● **Increasing co-ordination between health and education specialists** within development agencies in order to improve the intersectoral linkages between health and education programmes.

3. Food security, nutrition and health

Hunger and malnutrition are among the most devastating problems facing the world today. Although food security has improved in developing countries in the last 30 years, there has been a slowdown in the reduction of hunger in the 1990s. While the total number of undernourished people has declined (especially in China), in most countries the numbers have increased.[3] The international community is now committed to halving, by 2015, the proportion of people who suffer from hunger.[4]

Key linkages with poverty and health

Malnutrition and food insecurity, obviously, have strong implications for health. Nearly 800 million people in developing countries are chronically hungry. Many live in conflict areas and more than 60% of them are women.[5] Although the large majority of hungry people live in rural areas, rapid urbanisation contributes to increasing poverty and food insecurity in large towns and cities. *Hunger and malnutrition increase vulnerability to disease* and premature death, and reduce people's ability to earn a livelihood, not least through cultivation and generating an income. Malnutrition is both a major cause and effect, and a key indicator, of poverty and lack of development. Moreover, a failure to treat the underlying causes of malnutrition and their consequences undermines the impact of other efforts to improve health, while ill health itself reduces the ability of the body to absorb nutrients from food.

Malnutrition affects one in three people worldwide, especially the poor and vulnerable. Sixty per cent of annual deaths among children under five are associated with being underweight, while 161 million children are stunted in their linear growth. *Iodine deficiency* is the biggest single preventable cause of brain damage and mental retardation. *Iron deficiency anaemia* is second among leading causes of disability and may be a contributing factor in 20% of all maternal deaths. *Vitamin A deficiency* causes irreversible blindness and deaths among millions of children every year.[6]

Recommendations to development agencies

Agricultural development is essential to poverty reduction and improved food security. Development agencies play a major role in increasing agricultural output and stimulating rural development by supporting partner country strategies to increase the income-earning capacity of family farmers, generate rural employment, develop the rural non-farm economy, and enhance the availability and quality of the food produced. However, urbanisation is contributing to a blurring of the boundaries between rural and urban areas so that the poor in rural areas are increasingly likely to take up employment in small towns, engage in seasonal activities in urban areas, and send remittances that supplement rural incomes.[7] This calls for appropriate policy interventions that also address urban food insecurity, which is on the increase.

Hunger is related more to the availability of household income than to the availability of food. Improving food security is therefore essentially a question of managing access to food or increasing purchasing power. Supporting land-tenure reform, where politically feasible, can go a long way in helping to reduce poverty and increase food security. Other strategies that could be supported by development agencies include:[8]

- **The promotion of inclusiveness:** increasing incomes of the poorest groups, particularly for women, is likely to have a significant impact on reducing malnutrition.[9] Promoting empowerment by making institutions more responsive to the requirements of the poor, particularly women and marginalised groups, and by removing barriers that exclude individuals from economic and social opportunities on the basis of gender, social class, or ethnicity should be a priority.

- **Investment in rural projects:** irrigation, improved roads, and telecommunications projects can reduce the vulnerability of poor people in rural areas. During economic crises, governments can provide employment in public works programmes, which generally allow employment opportunities for poor people willing to take advantage of wages slightly below market rates. The value to the poor of such programmes is measured not only in terms of income support but also through benefits they receive from the infrastructure created.

- **Development of social safety nets:** these can benefit the poor and vulnerable just above the poverty line to prevent them from slipping into poverty. Although targeting and administering such programmes can be difficult, targeted food security programmes are generally more cost-effective than generalised food subsidies. In most situations, cash transfers or the provision of vouchers allow recipients to purchase the food they require through normal market channels. Transfers can be made part of broader programmes aimed at the nutrition of vulnerable children and pregnant women.

- **Management of disaster and conflict:** efforts to prevent disaster or resolve conflict rapidly can reduce the effects of famine and malnutrition.

Though increased incomes are essential, it has been shown that countries implementing direct nutrition interventions have been more successful in reducing malnutrition.[10] Targeted nutritional programmes depend on improved access to effective health services with health programmes for both mothers and children. Improving health programmes in schools will also provide further avenues for health education and nutritional programmes. Approaches targeting groups with the highest prevalence of malnutrition and hunger that should be supported include:

- **Designing special programmes for infants and children**, including the promotion of breastfeeding, supplementary feeding, immunisation, and the treatment of diarrhoea, respiratory infections, and malaria; *for women and adolescent girls*: nutritional supplements during pregnancy and breastfeeding such as iron, folic acid, iodised salt, food supplementation, and micronutrient-rich foods. Malaria and HIV/AIDS prevention and treatment is also particularly important.

- **Preventing micronutrient deficiencies** by designing and managing effective programmes for pre-school children and pregnant women to ensure sufficient intake of iodine, vitamin A and iron. Fortification of foods and micronutrients is also vital. The best known example globally is the iodisation of salt.

- **Ensuring appropriate child-feeding practices** by developing comprehensive national policies that ensure all health services protect, promote and support exclusive breastfeeding for six months.[11]

- **Managing nutrition during emergencies, conflict or disaster** for refugees, internally displaced people or other vulnerable groups. Nutritional programmes must be closely linked to priority health programmes such as immunisation and treatment for infectious diseases. *Emergency food aid* can save lives and protect health in such acute crises. Food aid can also be useful as targeted assistance to highly food-insecure people in situations of poorly functioning or fragile markets and serious institutional weakness.

4. Poverty, health and the environment

Estimates suggest that at least 25% of the global burden of disease may be attributed to environmental conditions.[12] This section focuses on two areas where the poverty-health-environment links are particularly strong – water and sanitation, and air pollution – and where sectoral policies ought to be assessed and improved to maximise opportunities for health promotion and protection. However, policy makers need also to consider other environmental hazards that may have a disproportionate impact on the health of the poor. Poor people are often subject, in their homes and workplaces, to exposure to toxic pollutants from sources including waste disposal sites and incinerators. Poor health status increases a person's vulnerability to the impact of toxic chemicals. It is important to have a healthy and safe work environment and a coherent policy for the safe use of chemicals, including their production, handling, storage, and disposal.[13]

4.1. *Water and sanitation*

Key linkages with poverty and health

The targets of halving the proportion of people living without sustainable access to safe water by 2015 and halving the proportion of people without access to basic sanitation adopted by the international community reflect the importance of improved access to water and sanitation to poverty reduction.[14]

Almost 1.2 billion people lack access to safe drinking water; twice that number lack adequate sanitation.[15] Inadequate water quality leads to the transmission of such diseases as diarrhoea, cholera, trachoma, and onchocercosis. Scabies and trachoma depend on the quantity of water available while stagnant water is a breeding ground for the vectors transmitting malaria and schistosomosis.[16] Access to adequate quantities of water is also essential for food production, which in turn improves nutrition, health and people's ability to withstand and recover from diseases. Lack of sanitation increases the transmission of excreta-related illnesses, including certain faecal-oral diseases such as cholera, soil-transmitted helminths (among them roundworms and hookworms), and water-based helminths (which cause, for example, schistosomosis). In addition, the contamination of water (and food) by pesticides and toxic chemicals such as mercury, lead and arsenic causes millions of cases of poisoning each year.[17]

The majority of people affected by these diseases are poor. Most of the resulting deaths are among children under five and are concentrated in poorest households and communities. According to one estimate, at any one time half of the urban population is suffering from one or more of the diseases associated with the provision of water and sanitation.[18] During conflicts and emergencies, people are even more vulnerable to water- and sanitation-related diseases.

Women are disproportionately affected. In rural areas, women spend many hours daily collecting and carrying water over long distances while in urban areas, women wait in queues for water from wells and standpipes. The carrying of water leads to chronic back pain, frequent miscarriages and uterine prolapse. Caring for sick family members and handling soiled clothes are particularly hazardous when water supplies are limited and sanitation insufficient, and women's responsibility for the disposal of waste exposes them to disease. The provision of sanitation is important for women not only for their physical health but also for their safety and dignity. In many cultures, women and girls can defecate only outside and after dark, which causes physical discomfort, serious illness and exposes them to the risk of sexual abuse. A lack of sanitation facilities in schools, furthermore, is a large contributing factor to preventing girls from attending school, increasingly so when they begin menstruation.

Recommendations to development agencies

The targets for access to safe water and sanitation will be achieved only through the concerted action of national governments in partnership with communities, civil society, the private sector and international development agencies. Governments are responsible for improving the frameworks for integrated water resource management (IWRM). These involve designing and implementing the policies that determine priorities, allocate water between uses, set prices, regulate private-sector providers, develop appropriate legal and financial instruments and ensure access to water especially for the poor. IWRM must be based on the understanding that the overall availability of water resources is fixed though population growth, increased food demand and an expanding industrial sector, will mean that demand for water will continue to rise.

Development agencies can play a role in ensuring that poor people's interests are reflected in these frameworks as well as strengthening the links between sectoral policies, health outcomes and poverty reduction strategies. They can also encourage governments to recognise the importance of involving communities, especially women, in the management and financing of water and sanitation systems. Development agencies can help build capacity in key government institutions. Specific areas of focus could include:

- **Improved data on access to, use of, and demand for water and sanitation** to facilitate planning and management and help ensure the sustainable availability of safe drinking water for poor people.

- **The development of an appropriate approach to financing water supplies** – not least the use of cost recovery and subsidies – that covers recurrent costs while protecting access for poor people.

- **Clearer recognition of the potential role of the private sector** in managing or expanding water and sanitation services through public-private partnerships with a range of private-sector entities, among them NGOs and civil society groups which are service providers in some countries and which have a strong poverty focus. In addition, the role of those private-sector organisations involved in small-scale water and sanitation provision, on which many poor people are dependent, is insufficiently understood. In countries where the legal and policy environment is weak, development agencies can help strengthen capacity for the beneficial regulation of the private sector.

- **Collaboration between environmental and public health authorities** within local authorities and international agencies on an integrated approach to water supply, sanitation, drainage, community education, and hygiene practices that emphasises the links between water, sanitation, health and poverty. Making health analysis an integral part of all environmental assessment procedures by government and development agencies can sharpen attention to these links.

- **Supporting the development of local capacity** to monitor water quality, the extent of any contamination, and the impact on health.

- **Promoting education in health and hygiene** to help stimulate demand for improved sanitation. Formal and non-formal education is an important vehicle for locally designed health- and hygiene-promotion programmes, a key component of effective interventions to improve water and sanitation. Hygiene behaviour, such as handling food with unwashed hands, can provide a substantial risk to health even where access to water has been improved, and many programmes have failed because insufficient attention was given to the local context.

Development agencies also need to help fill the resource gap if the water and sanitation targets are to be met. Estimates of needs vary significantly and further work is needed to develop more accurate estimates of the global financial requirements to meet the water- and sanitation-related targets.[19] The volume of resources required is likely to mean that in addition to public and private financing, development assistance will also be necessary.

4.2. Indoor and outdoor air pollution

Air pollution, indoors and out, is a major problem that affects the health of poor people disproportionately. Poverty leads to a dependence on cheap traditional fuels for cooking and heating which combines with unventilated, overcrowded accommodation to cause indoor pollution. In addition, in urban areas poor people live close to highly polluting industries and transport networks, with predictable effects on their health.

Indoor air pollution

Key linkages with poverty and health

Around 3 billion people are exposed to indoor air pollution from the use of traditional fuels for household energy. Poor households in sub-Saharan Africa and Asia rely mostly on biomass or kerosene because of cost; only the more affluent households use gas or electricity. Indoor air pollution causes an estimated 2 million deaths a year, mostly in developing countries.[20] It primarily affects the poor in rural areas but exposure is rising among urban populations.

Recommendations to development agencies

A number of interventions have been effective in reducing the impact of indoor air pollution, and yet development agency support for programmes has been limited. The success of these interventions depends not only on access to technology but also on decentralised management of programmes and training, combined with community involvement and ownership.[21] Development agencies should build on evaluations and support efforts for further replication of the interventions listed below in order to reach more poor people.

- **The most significant reduction in indoor air pollution comes from increasing access to improved cooking stoves**, which reduce particulate emissions from traditional fuels. Extensive improved stove programmes have been developed in China (reaching 120 million people) and India. Evaluation of such programmes has demonstrated considerable gains. Apart from the economic value of saving on fuel, cost-benefit analysis has shown that health improvements have produced further savings of around USD 25 to USD 100 per stove per year.[22]

- **Increasing access to cleaner fuel**, by increasing the supply and distribution of fuels such as kerosene.

- **Modifying the home environment to improve ventilation,** for example, cooking windows can reduce indoor carbon-monoxide levels.

- **Programmes to change behaviour,** such as improving understanding of the link between pollution and ill health and encouraging children to be kept away from smoke during peak cooking times.

Outdoor air pollution

Key linkages with poverty and health

Approximately 1.5 billion people are exposed to severe urban air pollution, the majority of them in developing countries. The most polluted cities are found in the developing world, among them Beijing, Cairo and Lagos where children regularly experience levels of air pollution 2 to 8 times above the maximum WHO guidelines on exposure. The burden of ill health caused by pollution in combination with sulphur dioxide is responsible for 4 to 5 million new cases of chronic bronchitis annually. Emissions from fossil fuel combustion and transportation are responsible for almost 90% of emissions in urban areas. Inadequate regulation, rapid urbanisation, the proximity of industries to residential areas, and high population density exacerbate the degree of exposure of poor people.

Recommendations to development agencies

Addressing the health impact of urban air pollution is complex. Technical, legal and economic instruments are being successfully used to control pollution in some countries though capacity to develop the legal, institutional and regulatory frameworks may be limited. Support from development agencies to strengthen the capacity to develop these frameworks is needed.[23] Major cities in China and India are increasing their use of cleaner energy, such as hydro power plants, solar panels and wind energy. In transport, Phnom Penh and Harare have introduced incentives for cycling, and Manila has increased fuel taxes and built a light railway, thus decreasing petrol consumption by 43% over ten years.

Development agencies should work together with partner countries to promote multisectoral energy policies that combine both economic and regulatory approaches and are based on collaboration between public and private sectors and civil society.[24] They should include:

- **Supporting capacity development in the management of air quality**, involving the use of economic instruments, managing fuel quality and pricing, and studying the impact of air pollution on health.

- **Shifting towards using modern energy sources and achieving higher energy efficiency**.

- **Investing in capacity building** for the management and planning of energy resources.

5. Violence and injuries as a public health issue

Violence is among the leading causes of death worldwide for people aged 15-44 years with over 90% of deaths from violence taking place in developing countries.[25] In 2000, an estimated 1.6 million people died as a result of violence: collective (death and injury resulting from war and related large-scale violent conflict), interpersonal and self-inflicted. The impact of conflict both on the health of the poor and on health services is addressed in Chapter 2, Section 3. In addition to violence, road traffic crashes are a major cause of death and injury in developing countries accounting for nearly 90% of worldwide traffic-related deaths.[26,27]

People with the lowest socio-economic status are at most risk of violence, and the risk is increased by factors related to poverty, such as bad housing, lack of education and unemployment. Statistically, for example, poorer women are more at risk of violence from their partners, and the young in poor communities are more likely to be involved in violence. Fatal violence, particularly of income earners, increases the risk of impoverishment and an increased dependency ratio. Poverty reduces the likelihood of access to health services, and injuries lead to reduced productivity and loss of income.

A public health approach to violence and injuries emphasises prevention. This section takes two examples – interpersonal violence and road traffic injuries – to highlight the impact on the health of poor people and the importance of multisectoral interventions.

5.1. *Interpersonal violence*

Key linkages with poverty and health

Interpersonal violence was responsible for at least 520 000 deaths in 2000, although that figure is an underestimate of the true burden that violence imposes because non-fatal violence is largely under-reported and heavily stigmatised. Surveys indicate nonetheless that *poor women and girls are especially vulnerable to physical, sexual and psychological violence*, including rape, genital mutilation, forced marriage and prostitution, widow abuse and the neglect of elderly women, and murder (of both female infants and young women). Two million women and girls are subjected to genital mutilation annually, while thousands are killed by their relatives to protect the "family honour". In addition, an estimated 2 million girls are part of the international sex trade each year. The evidence also suggests that after adjusting for sex and age, the risk of being a victim of violence is significantly higher for young people from low socio-economic classes. In developing countries, women lose an estimated 5% of their healthy life years as a consequence of rape and domestic violence.

The direct consequences of interpersonal violence range from injury to death; the effects are compounded when women are denied access to health care. Being a victim of violence also increases women's risk of future ill health from a variety of diseases and conditions. In particular, sexual violence can lead to unwanted pregnancy and sexually transmitted diseases including HIV, and violence by partners accounts for a substantial proportion of maternal mortality. Women victims of abuse are more likely to be long-term users of health services, thereby increasing health care costs. In addition, several studies have estimated the economic burden of violence created by interpersonal violence and its health consequences. In Nicaragua, for example, female victims of domestic abuse earned 46% less than their unaffected counterparts, even after controlling for other factors that could affect earnings.

Recommendations for development agencies

Interpersonal violence can be substantially reduced.[28] Creating safe and healthy communities requires multisectoral commitment from governments and communities to build awareness of the problem, to promote the design and testing of prevention programmes, and to share lessons learned. Development agencies can support the efforts of partner countries for:

- **An adequately resourced public health approach that focuses on prevention** and contributes to reducing violence through the development of national plans and policies, the facilitation of data collection, and the development of multisectoral partnerships.

- **Integrating violence prevention into social, health and education policies.**

- **Training for health-sector staff** who have a key role to play in providing health care, counselling and psychosocial support for the victims of violence as well as in detecting signs of violent incidents.

5.2. Road traffic injuries

Key linkages with poverty and health

Road traffic crashes cause the death of over a million people annually in developing countries; worldwide, 10 million people are injured or disabled.[29] The poor are at more risk of road traffic injuries, particularly as vulnerable road-users such as pedestrians, bicyclists, those on motorised two-wheelers, passengers in mini-buses. These categories make up some 90% of fatalities in developing countries. It is estimated that by 2020 road traffic crashes will be the third leading cause of the burden of disease worldwide. *In developing countries, road traffic injuries are a leading cause of mortality and morbidity; they are responsible for an immense burden on national health systems.* According to one study, those injured in crashes can occupy up to 25% of hospital beds at any one time, cause major economic and social consequences, and are a drain on limited national resources.[30]

The mix of unsafe vehicles, poor road infrastructure and inefficient law enforcement sets the scene for an unprecedented confluence of risks on the road. Inadequate trauma care, poor public health infrastructure, and limited pre-hospital care exacerbate injuries, prolong the need for treatment, and/or result in disabling sequela.[31] Injuries are concentrated in those under 45 years of age and tend to affect productivity severely, particularly among the lowest income groups who are most exposed to risk. Loss of an income earner, the substantial cost of prolonged medical care, particularly when administered in hospital, and loss of household income because of disability can precipitate poverty in the affected household. The ripples of this loss can be felt by the extended family and by informal community support systems that are often called upon to contribute towards medical bills and care for the bereaved family.[32]

Recommendations to development agencies

More attention must be paid to making the environment safer for those not using a car but who are at considerable risk of being hit by one. Since the types of road traffic crashes in developing countries differ considerably from those in the developed world, prevention strategies cannot simply be exported from developed countries. Effective traffic injury prevention programmes are being implemented in some countries, often as pilot projects.

DAC GUIDELINES AND REFERENCE SERIES: POVERTY AND HEALTH – ISBN 92-64-10018-0 – © OECD, WHO 2003

Development co-operation agencies can assist prevention by supporting the evaluation and replication of effective programmes, including:

- **The development of a multisectoral approach,** for example, improving data collection through support for injury surveillance systems in hospitals, health clinics and police stations. Groups involving health, police, transport and education sectors should design interventions based on data analysis. Possible interventions include the promulgation and enforcement of regulations such as those requiring the use of seat belts and preventing the running of traffic lights, and laws governing the wearing of helmets and the consumption of alcohol.

- **The use of health and education channels to raise awareness of the problem** and promote safety focusing particularly on children and vulnerable road users.

- **The improvement of roadways** and other engineering measures such as roundabouts and bridges for pedestrians, which can reduce crashes.

- **The development of appropriate financial risk-management systems to protect low-income households** from catastrophic health expenditure after road traffic crashes.

Notes

1. Investment in basic education for girls has among the highest returns of all economic development programmes. Educated women are more likely to send their children to school, have higher earnings, are more likely to participate in society and help protect the environment, and have fewer and healthier children. Societies that deny education to girls experience poorer health and poorer economic growth.

2. ICT may be a valuable tool in health education and can increase the use of community radio, broadcast media, telecoms, etc. for the wide dissemination of health messages.

3. FAO (UN Food and Agriculture Organization) (2001), FAO Warns Further Slowdown in Hunger Reduction – In most Developing Countries the Number of Hungry even Increased. *Press Release 01/69*. Accessible at www.fao.org/waicent/ois/press_ne/presseng/2001/pren0169.htm

4. Two of the indicators for measuring performance are the prevalence of underweight children (under five years of age) and the proportion of the population below minimum level of dietary energy consumption.

5. ACC/SCN and IFPRI (2000), *Fourth Report on the World Nutrition Situation*, UN Sub-Committee on Nutrition. See also ACC/SCN (2002), *Nutrition: A Foundation for Development*, ACC/SCN, Geneva.

6. UNICEF (2001), *Vitamin A Deficiency*. Accessible at www.childinfo.org/eddb/vita_a/index.htm

7. World Bank (2002), *Reaching the Rural Poor*, World Bank. Accessible at http://wbln0018.worldbank.org/ESSD/rdv/vta.nsf/Gweb/Strategy

8. *Ibid.*

9. See Smith, L. and L. Haddad (2000), Overcoming Child Malnutrition in Developing Countries: Past Achievements and Future Choices. *2020 Brief No. 64*, IFPRI. Accessible at *www.ifpri.org/2020/briefs/number64.htm*

10. Alderman, H. *et al.* (2001), Reducing Child Malnutrition: How Far Does Income Growth Take Us? *CREDIT Research Paper No. 01/05*, University of Nottingham. Accessible at www.nottingham.ac.uk/economics/credit/research/papers/cp.01.05.pdf

11. WHO (2002), *Resolution World Health Assembly 55.25 Global Strategy on Infant and Young Child Feeding*. It also emphasises the role of community attitudes, which can be promoted through mother and child-friendly communities in hospitals and workplaces, and implementation of the International Code of Marketing of Breast-milk Substitutes and subsequent WHA resolutions.

12. WEHAB Working Group (2002a), *A Framework for Action on Health and the Environment*, United Nations. Accessible at www.johannesburgsummit.org/html/documents/summit_docs/wehab_papers/wehab_health.pdf

13. See the Chemicals Convention (C170, 1990) of the International Labour Organization (ILO) and the ILO Safety and Health in Agriculture Convention (C176, 2001) and other related conventions and recommendations on health and safety. Accessible at *www.ilo.org*

14. See MDG Goal 7, target 10, and the Plan of Implementation of the World Summit on Sustainable Development (advanced unedited text, 4 September 2002).

15. Sanitation is the safe management of waste. Hospitals and health facilities are themselves a source of hazardous waste, which can be environmentally damaging and impact on the health of poor people.

16. Diarrhoeal diseases cause 3.3 million premature deaths per year, trachoma blinds 6-9 million people per year, and schistosomosis affects 200 million people annually. See WELL (1999), *DFID Guidance Manual on Water Supply and Sanitation Programmes*, WELL Resource Centre. Accessible at *www.lboro.ac.uk/well/index.htm*

17. WEHAB Working Group (2002a) *op. cit.*

18. WHO (1996), *Creating Health Cities in the 21st Century* Background Paper prepared for the Dialogue on Health in Human Settlements for Habitat II, WHO, Geneva.

19. WEHAB Working Group (2002b), *A Framework for Action on Water and Sanitation*. Accessible at www.johannesburgsummit.org/html/documents/summit_docs/wehab_papers/ wehab_water_sanitation.pdf

20. WEHAB Working Group (2002a) *op. cit.*

21. Kammen, D.M. (1995), Cookstoves for the Developing World, *Scientific American*, July, pp. 64-67.

22. *Ibid.*

23. WEHAB Working Group (2002a), *op. cit.*

24. WEHAB Working Group (2002a), *op. cit.*

25. Most of the statistics on violence are from WHO (2002), *World Report on Violence and Health*, WHO, Geneva. Accessible at *www5.who.int/violence_injury_prevention/main.cfm?p=0000000682*

26. Murray, C.J.L. and A.D. Lopez (1996), *Global Health Statistics: A Compendium of Incidence, Prevalence and Mortality Estimates for over 200 Conditions*, Harvard University Press, Boston.

27. Krug, E. (ed.) (1999), *Injury A Leading Cause of the Global Burden of Disease*, WHO, Geneva.

28. These recommendations are derived from the WHO (2002), *World Report on Violence and Health*, WHO, Geneva and the experience of the German Agency for Technical Co-operation (GTZ).

29. Murray, C.J.L. and A.D. Lopez (1996), *op. cit.*

30. Andrews, C.N., O.C. Kobusingye and R. Lett (1999), "Road Traffic Accident Injuries in Kampala", *East African Medical Journal*; Vol. 76, No. 4: pp. 189-194; Hijar, M., C. Carrillo, M. Flores, R. Anaya and V. Lopez (2000), "Risk Factors in Highway Traffic Accidents: A Case Control Study", *Accident Analysis and Prevention*, Vol. 32: pp. 703-709.

31. Nantulya, V. and M. Reich (2002), "The Neglected Epidemic: Road Traffic Injuries in Developing Countries", *British Medical Journal*; 324: 1139-1141.

32. Jamison, D.T. (1996), "Investing in Health Research and Development", *Report of the Ad Hoc Committee on World Health Organization Health Research Relating to Future Intervention Options*, WHO, Geneva.

DAC GUIDELINES AND REFERENCE SERIES: POVERTY AND HEALTH – ISBN 92-64-10018-0 – © OECD, WHO 2003

ISBN 92-64-10018-0
DAC Guidelines and Reference Documents
Poverty and Health
© OECD, WHO 2003

Chapter 4

Frameworks and Instruments for Health Programming and Monitoring

Abstract. Development agencies should support pro-poor health policies that are owned by partner countries. To do this, they rely upon a range of development co-operation instruments and approaches: policy dialogue, budget support, sectoral programmes, projects, technical co-operation, debt relief and global health initiatives. To be effective, these instruments should be deployed within nationally owned frameworks such as the Poverty Reduction Strategy (PRS). Supplementing this, a national health-sector programme may be the appropriate framework for negotiating and supporting policies likely to improve the health of poor people. The sector-wide approach (SWAp) aims specifically to strengthen co-ordination in support of improved government-led health policies and increasingly relies on government for management, implementation and funding procedures. As part of their efforts to support the implementation of PRS and health-sector programmes, development agencies should assist partner countries in monitoring health system performance and health outcomes and the extent to which they are pro-poor.

1. Introduction

The commitment to support the health-related MDGs calls for a long-term relationship with partner countries. Development agencies should focus on building partnerships in which they can *support pro-poor health policies owned by the country and co-ordinate with other bilateral and multilateral organisations* to ensure consistency between approaches.

To this end, development agencies may rely upon a range of co-operation instruments and approaches: policy dialogue, budget support, sectoral programmes, projects, technical co-operation, debt relief and global health initiatives. *If these instruments are to be effective, they should be deployed within commonly agreed frameworks* that help to set priorities and focus the purpose of interventions. The overarching framework is the national poverty reduction strategy (PRS) discussed below. Supplementing this, a health-sector programme may be the appropriate framework for negotiating and supporting priorities specific to that sector, and particularly for engaging in a dialogue on the policies and interventions likely to improve the health of poor people. The sector-wide approach (SWAp) is discussed in this context since it aims specifically to strengthen co-ordination in support of improved government-led health policies and increasingly relies on government for management, implementation and funding procedures.

2. Development co-operation instruments for pro-poor health

Each development co-operation instrument has advantages and disadvantages. They should be used in combinations that fit national conditions. The issue currently under debate is primarily balance among instruments, overall and for each development agency.

- **As the mode of delivery moves "upstream" towards programme aid and budget support**, the opportunity arises for a shift to approaches that are led by governments, based on domestically developed policies and rooted in national systems and procedures. The further upstream the mode of delivery, however, the more the development agency should be convinced that there are: i) consensus on government policies and resource allocation for health and poverty reduction; ii) capacity and commitment to carry out the programme; iii) financial and performance-management systems to ensure that resources are spent as agreed in health-sector expenditure frameworks; and iv) adequate reporting and monitoring mechanisms to track expected health outcomes for the poor. Upstream budget support addresses fundamental policy and allocation issues and requires a significant investment in capacity building and policy reform. As such, it needs a long-term commitment by development partners if it is to have an impact on health outcomes.

- **Downstream project support** can yield immediate measurable benefits for targeted vulnerable groups but cannot always address systemic issues in health service delivery or the cross-cutting and deeply embedded problems of poverty. Agencies must ensure that projects are integrated into the health-sector programme and enhance local

DAC GUIDELINES AND REFERENCE SERIES: POVERTY AND HEALTH – ISBN 92-64-10018-0 – © OECD, WHO 2003

capacity to plan and implement health service delivery. Large numbers of small projects, with separate missions and implementation arrangements, should be avoided; they tax the limited capacities of partner countries.

3. Poverty reduction strategies and health

The emphasis on poverty reduction promoted by processes such as developing Poverty Reduction Strategy Papers (PRSP)[1] could have considerable implications for the way that pro-poor health programmes are designed and funded. More broadly, PRSs could potentially provide an important framework for understanding the practical relationship between pro-poor health objectives and policies in other sectors. As suggested below, a number of challenges must be overcome if the potential of PRSs for promoting pro-poor health policies is to be realised. Development agencies, in particular, can support the following actions:

- **Involve health constituencies in PRS formulation and increase their capacity to influence policy-making.** Partner countries require time to lead, develop and own their poverty reduction strategies. Consultation across government and with civil society should be an intrinsic part of this process. Within government, PRS development is typically led by a small group based in the ministries of finance, economic affairs or planning, or in the President's office. This step represents a welcome "upgrading" of poverty issues to the most senior tiers of government, but it should be balanced by mechanisms which ensure that sectoral ministries play a full role in PRS development. Experience from PRSPs[2] suggests that health ministries in particular have not yet contributed in any large measure to their overall development, and, in some cases, even to the health content. Development agencies should help increase their capacity to do so. They should also support efforts to reflect the health concerns of civil society (parliament, local government, community organisations, advocacy groups for women's health, trade unions, and the private sector) in policy choices and priorities.

- **Emphasise the causal links between better health and poverty reduction.** Most PRSs recognise health as a dimension of poverty, and many make direct or indirect reference to the importance of improved health to development and growth. Indeed, health appears as a key strategic component in the majority of PRSPs.[3] Yet most PRSs do not explore the causal links in sufficient depth, even allowing for lack of space.

- **Improve links with health-sector programmes and gender policies.** So far, the linkages between poverty reduction strategies, health-sector programmes and gender policies have been weak. The PRS has limited space for detailed sectoral analysis and is often too unspecific to prioritise clearly or force hard decisions. In addition, there is often a mismatch of targets, or key targets in one framework are not carried forward into another. Specific contributions from agencies to assist partner countries in making explicit links between health, gender and PRS include:

  ❖ Ensure that PRS objectives and targets are reflected in health-sector programmes and in national policy frameworks on gender equality and vice-versa, with robust strategies for achieving proposed outcomes.

  ❖ Encourage the use of analysis specific to the health sector to inform PRS and build capacity in health ministries for gender and poverty analysis.[4]

  ❖ Use the PRS framework to encourage links between health and other ministries, including women's ministries and departments responsible for water, sanitation, education and nutrition in order to develop multisectoral strategies that are known to have a major impact on poor people's health (see Chapter 3).

- **Explore the added value of the PRS from a health perspective.** While PRSs cannot and should not replace existing health-sector programmes, they do provide an important opportunity to take a fresh look at health programmes to ensure that health outcomes improve for poor people. Development agencies should work with governments to use the PRS process as a first step in reassessing existing health strategies from a poverty perspective rather than simply drawing out the perceived pro-poor components of existing national health programmes.

4. Health-sector programmes and their effectiveness in reducing poverty

Health-sector programmes provide a key framework to channel development co-operation in support of national health policies. Health-sector programmes can be supported by the full range of aid instruments, from projects to support of the overall budget in which the health programme is included. Health-sector programmes allow agencies to engage in a dialogue on the policies and interventions likely to improve the health of the poor.

4.1. Focusing health-sector programmes on pro-poor objectives

In order to meet the health needs and priorities of the poor, sector programmes require an explicit emphasis on pro-poor objectives and approaches. This focus can be achieved in several ways that development agencies should emphasise:

- **Decision-making on policies to improve poor people's health should rely on rigorous poverty and gender analysis.**[5] For example, there should be a deeper understanding of what services the poor use and why, how gender affects access and impact of services, and how funds are channelled to meet priorities. Agencies should support capacity development in this area both inside the line ministry and in external institutions, ensure that poverty and gender analysis are built into sector-planning and review cycles, and encourage open dialogue on the results. Ownership by national governments should not exclude discussion about issues that may not yet be a priority for governments, such as pro-poor health and gender equality. Policy dialogue can be informed by international priorities, such as those agreed at UN conferences.[6]

- **Responsive health systems presuppose a dynamic dialogue between policy makers and beneficiaries.** A sector programme may not always provide for stakeholder participation. But agencies must ensure that consultation and participation continue throughout the health-sector planning and review cycles, both through existing structures (local government, NGOs, community organisations, trade unions and women's groups) and through innovative approaches designed to access the opinions of the poor, and hard-to-reach and under-represented groups.

- **The sector programme should include those policies and services that most affect the poor directly** and poor women in particular (*e.g.* primary health care, essential obstetric care) as well as those for which the funding directly affects the overall resources available for services for the poor. This would include, for example, funding for teaching hospitals and also for HIV/AIDS prevention, care and support programmes. Ideally, the sector programme should move towards comprehensive coverage of key areas of provision for the poor, namely public health programmes, health services, health financing and social protection (as discussed in Chapters 2 and 3).

- **Coverage should not be limited to the public sector – it should also encompass the private sector and NGOs.** The contribution of the private health sector often requires redefinition of the relationship with government (see Chapter 2). Development agencies may wish to encourage contractual forms of relationship by redirecting some NGO funding through government systems. But agencies should consider the impact on piloting and innovation, often areas of excellence among NGOs, and on the political acceptability of funding services for minority or special interest groups.

- **Global Health Initiatives should be integrated into the sector programme.** GHIs provide significant funding to programmes that may improve the health of the poor (see Chapter 2). But their discrete policy stances and vertical funding modalities have made integration into national health planning processes challenging. Development agencies should ensure that global initiatives do not distort country ownership or the growing ability to plan and finance without earmarking. This safeguard can be achieved by i) ensuring that GHIs are included in the PRS process, national health strategies and Medium-Term Expenditure Frameworks (MTEF); ii) addressing areas of inconsistency between GHI contributions and national accountability structures, making use of common procedures for financing, monitoring and evaluation; and iii) linking in-country co-ordination of GHI with ministry of health management structures, annual health-sector reviews and monitoring arrangements.

- **The sector programme should operate within well-designed and managed decentralised systems.** Decentralisation is seen in many countries, in health as in other areas, as the key to providing accessible services that are responsive to the needs of the poor. But sector programmes are negotiated with central government and for consultation with local authorities they usually rely on existing institutional arrangements, which may be weak, lacking in accountability and unrepresentative. Development agencies can help ensure that sector programmes support decentralisation and increase local capacity to deliver appropriate services.

4.2. Taking a sector-wide approach to health programming and delivery

Sector-wide approaches (SWAps) in health merit attention because they are relatively new and aim to strengthen co-ordination. The sector-wide approach is a health-sector programme, as discussed above, in which i) the partner government clearly leads and owns the programme, and ii) there is a common effort by external partners in support of that programme, including through providing all or a major share of funding for the sector in support of the government's unified policy and expenditure programme. Over time, some SWAps progress towards using government procedures for implementation and the disbursement of funds. In practice, most programmes are in the process of drawing diverse channels of funding into the programme, making the coverage of the sector more comprehensive, bringing ongoing projects into line with sector priorities, developing common procedures, and placing increased reliance on government for management.

Where SWAps are appropriate, they can help to promote greater local involvement, accountability and capacity in partner countries. SWAps are no panacea, though, and are indicated only when key preconditions can be largely met. The decision to take a SWAp must be made as a result of careful appraisal of conditions within the partner country, specifically the macro-economic, policy and institutional environment.

- **The environment in which a SWAp may be appropriate to promote pro-poor health, is one in which:**

  ❖ The partner country has developed a PRS and is committed to implementing it.

  ❖ Development agencies and government can reach agreement on policies and priorities to promote a pro-poor health approach.

  ❖ There is a supportive macro budget environment, and confidence among all parties that agreed government resources will be available for promoting a pro-poor health approach.

  ❖ Accounting as well as fiduciary arrangements are transparent.

  ❖ The external contribution to the health sector is large enough for co-ordination to be a problem, and for government to be willing to let development agencies influence policy; government should see that leading on the management of combined development co-operation is more advantageous than brokering fragmented agency funding.

  ❖ There is a critical mass of development agencies with activities in the health sector prepared to harmonise approaches to management, monitoring, and, to some extent, funding arrangements.

In essence, a SWAp calls for a partnership in which government and development agencies change their relationships (to clearer government leadership). They interact more together in the formulation of policy, and less on the details of its implementation. This partnership should be premised on: creating an atmosphere of mutual trust and greater commitment; sharing responsibility for addressing problems; accepting joint accountability and relinquishing attribution; managing collectively, rather than agencies prescribing and administering each funded transaction; and accepting some increase in financial and institutional risk. These requirements present challenges to development agencies in terms of the investments they must make to promote ownership and accountability, build capacity within government, and to change their own practices to facilitate the development of a SWAp.

- **Promote country ownership and accountability.** Strong government ownership is a clear goal of the SWAp and essential if the government is going to take leadership for improving health and addressing poverty. The process of sector-wide integrated planning – moving from fragmented, stand-alone projects to a unified system – provides an important vehicle for increasing government ownership and control. It calls for agencies to step back from their previous practices of strong direction and concern with detailed implementation, and focus on the intended outputs and the broad orientations to achieve them. Agencies have legitimate concerns as to how their funds are used; they should be addressed by agreeing on performance indicators and building appropriate management systems, including the sector programme annual review process. New forms of partnerships to improve accountability are in place to facilitate ownership whilst ensuring performance, including earmarking of expenditure, graduated releases against agreed performance benchmarks, joint annual reviews, *aide-mémoires* with agreed implementation targets, and ground rules set out in "Memoranda of Understanding" and "Codes of Conduct".

● **Build capacity within government.** A key objective of the SWAp is capacity building within government – the capacity to own, lead, implement and sustain policy-making and implementation. It affords an opportunity to invest in the capacity of core government systems even beyond the ministry of health. Many of the principal problems that have stymied health ministries lie in other, more powerful departments. Agencies should therefore work with governments more broadly, to address such issues as staff appointments and performance, management, budgeting, accounting and procurement. They should also look beyond their technical remits and share investments in capacity, moving away from micro initiatives and being bold enough to tackle more fundamental issues. Inasmuch as the sector-wide approach removes agencies from the detail of project management, the partnership requires good dialogue on the larger policy issues.

● **Change the practices of development agencies.** Many agencies find that one of the biggest challenges to creating a conducive environment for a SWAp is in changing their behaviour and work practices. Supporting a SWAp requires agencies to take part in co-ordination, sign up to the sector strategy, accept a degree of harmonisation in reporting, move towards allowing government to take the lead in implementing ongoing projects, and participate in fungible funding modalities. When agencies retain their individual reporting and management systems, the SWAp cannot meet its full potential to increase ownership and capacity. A sector-wide approach must both satisfy agency accountability to their domestic constituents and increase partner governments' accountability to their populations for the external funds they receive. That requires more capacity to manage the use of the funds, and ownership of the results.

If SWAps are to be sustainable, development agencies will have to resist their own demands for immediate results. Progress may not be immediately recognisable in the traditional monitoring systems agencies use, where the emphasis is on short-term indicators. Yet the sector programme also requires built in, rigorous monitoring – used by partner governments as well as development agencies – that measures more than the mere processes (see next section).

The issue for development agencies is not whether to stop project support and move exclusively to SWAps, or to overall budget support. Rather, the challenge that development agencies face, individually and as a group, is how to determine the right mix among the three – and between them and assistance coming through global programmes – at the country and global level. This is a topic that merits both ongoing attention and joint learning.

5. Measuring and monitoring progress

5.1. *Measuring health system performance and health outcomes*

As part of their efforts to implement PRSs and health-sector programmes, partner countries must measure health system performance and health outcomes and the extent to which they are pro-poor. On the one hand, the growing recognition of the role of policies and interventions outside the health sector to improve health, coupled with the move towards budget support in development co-operation, requires a focus on health outcomes. On the other hand, the performance of health systems has to be monitored from a pro-poor perspective, which calls for a range of indicators tracing inputs and processes.

Statistical systems are generally weak in partner countries. Many low-income countries lack functioning registration systems, and data on causes of death and the incidence of disease are often absent. For these countries, there are few baseline estimates against which the impact of health interventions can be measured. Furthermore, the lack of disaggregated data (by sex, income group, region) makes it difficult to capture the impact of policies and interventions – within and beyond the sector – on the health of the poor.

When data are available, they are often poorly managed and used. National planning and implementation systems have seldom developed an institutional culture of using data derived from management information systems to implement their programmes more effectively. Often, poverty data generated by the national statistics office or some other government department are not combined with health data generated by the ministry of health. Externally conducted information systems – such as Demographic and Health Surveys (DHS) and Living Standards Measurement Surveys (LSMS) – are able to fill these gaps only partially, since they are seldom integrated in the national health management information systems.

5.2. Adequate monitoring systems – meeting a hierarchy of need

Measuring the performance of health systems and pro-poor health outcomes requires a responsive information system that includes: i) an analysis of poverty and health determinants, including gender; ii) realistic quantitative targets and benchmarks (modelling); iii) base-line data; iv) policy and programme monitoring (input/output/outcome) with indicators developed at the planning stage; v) benefit incidence analysis; vi) impact evaluation; and vii) feedback mechanisms.

- **Partner countries require sound monitoring systems for a variety of purposes.** Information is necessary for evidence-based planning, accountability, advocacy, communication and resource mobilisation. Ministries of planning and finance require an overview of the performance of all sectors to justify budgets, to gauge the progress of the national PRS and to report against international obligations.

- **Monitoring systems ought to be able to reconcile national and international requirements and obligations.** The main objective should be to strengthen national data collection and analysis for local decision-making and for monitoring the implementation of the PRS and the health-sector programme. But countries also have international obligations – for example, to report on notifiable communicable diseases. Furthermore, there is increasing consensus on the importance of monitoring a few core indicators linked closely to the eight MDGs (with 18 targets and 48 indicators) and, specifically, to the three goals related to health as shown in Table 2. It will be important to ensure that monitoring of the MDGs in individual countries is integrated into existing monitoring systems.

5.3. Collaborative efforts to strengthen statistical and monitoring capacity

A major effort is necessary to strengthen statistical infrastructure and systems in support of pro-poor health. It is best provided through a co-ordinated approach integrated with the formulation, implementation and monitoring of poverty reduction strategies.

The gradual shift towards programme assistance and budget support has highlighted the gaps in existing monitoring systems. Many agencies are moving towards results-based assistance that links funding to specific improvements in health outcomes. New global health initiatives – such as the GAVI and the GFATM – emphasise the achievement of outcomes. It is important that these multiple monitoring systems are embedded in an effective country-led system and that perverse incentives – such as over-reporting of a disease burden in order to attract assistance or over-reporting of achievements to maintain funding – are avoided.

Table 2. **Health-related Millennium Development Goals**

Goals and Targets of the Millennium Declaration	Indicators for Monitoring Progress
Goal 4: Reduce child mortality	
Target 5: Reduce by two-thirds, between 1990 and 2015, the under-five mortality rate	• Under-five mortality rate • Infant mortality rate • Proportion of one-year-old children immunised against measles
Goal 5: Improve maternal health	
Target 6: Reduce by three-quarters, between 1990 and 2015, the maternal mortality ratio	• Maternal mortality ratio • Proportion of births attended by skilled health personnel
Goal 6: Combat HIV/AIDS, malaria and other diseases	
Target 7: Have halted by 2015 and begun to reverse the spread of HIV/AIDS	• HIV prevalence among 15/24 year-old pregnant women • Condom use rate of the contraceptive prevalence rate* • Number of children orphaned by HIV/AIDS
Target 8: Have halted by 2015 and begun to reverse the incidence of malaria and other major diseases	• Prevalence and death rates associated with malaria • Proportion of population in malaria risk areas using effective measures for malaria prevention and treatment • Prevalence and death rates associated with tuberculosis • Proportion of tuberculosis cases detected and cured under directly observed treatment, short-course (DOTS)
Goal 8: Develop a Global Partnership for Development	
Target 17: In co-operation with pharmaceutical companies, provide access to affordable essential drugs in developing countries	• Proportion of population with access to affordable, essential drugs on a sustainable basis

*   Among contraceptive methods, only condoms are effective in reducing HIV transmission. The contraceptive prevalence rate is also useful in tracking progress in other health, gender and poverty goals.
Source: World Bank (2002).

The PARIS21[7] Consortium, a partnership of policy makers, analysts and statisticians focuses specifically on strengthening statistical systems and on promoting, in the longer term, a culture of evidence-based policy-making and monitoring in all countries, with a focus on low-income countries. Its work will serve to improve transparency, accountability and the quality of governance.

Work to select appropriate indicators for monitoring the performance of health systems and pro-poor health outcomes has been initiated by a number of development agencies. DFID, for example, is leading a joint programme (over 2003–2009) with participation from the EC, World Bank, USAID and others to improve capacity to measure poverty and health, to monitor health system performance, and to evaluate PRS and health-sector reforms in achieving pro-poor health outcomes.

A core function of the WHO (which routinely reports health outcomes for all of its member States) is to help countries strengthen their health information systems. The WHO is in the process of carrying out a *World Health Survey* which aims to help countries fill crucial gaps in their health information systems. It also works on improving the validation process for indicators used in routine measurement by advocating five quality criteria for health information: validity, comparability across populations and countries, reliability, an audit trail, and validation in the country itself.

5.4. Principles to guide development co-operation in monitoring progress

In supporting efforts by partner countries to build effective monitoring systems and to measure progress towards improving the health of the poor, development agencies should consider the following guiding principles:

- **Where possible, use and build on what is in place.** Avoid creating parallel systems. Any effort should reinforce national capacity and country ownership. A number of countries where sector-wide approaches in health are in place (Ghana, Mozambique, Uganda) have already selected about 20 sector-wide indicators that provide a basis for monitoring health outcomes.[8]

- **Measuring health outcomes and monitoring health system performance are equally important.** While there is an increased focus on health outcomes, it is also necessary to monitor the extent to which health systems become pro-poor in terms of ensuring access, equity and fair financing. This includes the monitoring of such variables as the patterns in which health care is sought, willingness/ability to pay, utilisation by gender, efficiency, quality, financial accessibility and progress towards meeting the MDGs. New intermediate indicators are required to link health-sector processes to pro-poor health outcomes, and there is still considerable work required to ensure that suggested indicators can be measured in a reliable and comparable way.

- **Co-ordination, collaborative efforts and harmonisation of procedures are important.** Indicators in PRSs, health-sector programmes, in mid-term and annual plans, as well as in the country strategies of development agencies have to be consistent. Core global indicators and guidelines agreed by all agencies and parties should be used, and they should be focused on a limited number of relevant and practical variables. Information provided should meet the requirements of the policy process and the demands of good public administration. Indicators should be relevant, feasible to measure and able to track changes over time, and data collection should be inexpensive and involve no additional workload. The increasing trends towards results-based disbursement may, however, create perverse incentives in order to generate additional funding.

- **Invest in building national capacity in management information** within and outside the public sector. Facilitate joint working for performance assessment across government and civil society. All programmes should budget adequately for monitoring and evaluation (M&E) activities; this principle should preferably be built into the PRS process. The national health information system can be complemented by work contracted out to independent universities or other research institutions. In some countries, existing sentinel surveillance sites and population laboratories can be expanded and the potential benefits of special surveys (such as the DHS) can be maximised.

- **Accept a trade-off between statistical quality, completeness and the costs of collecting representative data.** Use proxy measures and build up an overall picture of progress from diverse and complementary data sources. Start with a few robust quantitative indicators and good qualitative process indicators. Countries will have to fund data systems in the medium to long term. A limited system focusing on a few core indicators will be more sustainable than a comprehensive system. In addition, not all the key data have to be measured each year, or even by the routine information system; intermittent monitoring is appropriate for some key variables.

Notes

1. National PRSPs are required in all low-income countries receiving concessional support from the World Bank and IMF. They provide channels for national and sectoral debt-relief expenditure and have the potential to increase external funding for poverty focused programmes.

2. WHO (2002), *Health in PRSPs – WHO Submission to World Bank/IMF Review of PRSPs*, December 2001.

3. WHO (2002), *PRSPs – Their Significance for Health*, STU/PRSP/02.1, October 2002.

4. Making use of material such as guidelines for gender assessment studies (micro/meso), gender checklists for institutional sector and organisational analyses (meso), guidelines for gender-aware budget analyses, reference material for gender and macro-economic sectoral analyses. World Bank (2002), *A Sourcebook for Poverty Reduction Strategies, Volume 1*. World Bank, Washington.

5. The DAC Working Party on Gender Equality has produced guidance on gender equality and SWAps emphasising the links between poverty, gender equality and instruments such as Medium-Term Expenditure Frameworks. In particular, it notes the need for sector programmes to: move towards comprehensive gender equality concepts; link integration of gender equality in the sector to national frameworks; carry out institution building and capacity building for gender equality; co-ordinate development agency support of gender equality in sector work. This is particularly needed in the health sector, where capacity in gender analysis is often weak. OECD (2002), *Gender Equality in Sector Wide Approaches: A Reference Guide*, Development Assistance Committee, OECD, Paris.

6. These include: The International Conference on Population and Development 1994, The World Summit for Social Development 1995, The Fourth World Conference on Women 1995, and The Millennium Summit 2000.

7. PARIS21 was launched at a meeting held in Paris in November 1999 at the initiative of the UN, OECD, World Bank, IMF and the EC in response to a UN ECOSOC resolution on indicators and statistical capacity building.

8. In Ghana there are 25 indicators measuring inputs, outputs and outcomes in terms of: access, quality, efficiency/effectiveness, partnership and financing. [See Accorsi, S. (2002), "*Measuring Health Sector Performance Through Indicators: Toward Evidence-Based Policy: A Review of the Experience of Performance Monitoring in the Framework of the Sector-Wide Approach in Ghana*". Unpublished Paper, European Commission, March 2002].

ISBN 92-64-10018-0
DAC Guidelines and Reference Documents
Poverty and Health
© OECD, WHO 2003

Chapter 5

Policy Coherence and Global Public Goods

Abstract.   *The health problems of the poor do not stop at national borders. A globalised world presents new risks to health and at the same time, it provides opportunities to prevent, treat or contain disease. Development agencies and partner countries should strengthen ways of working together globally. One way is to promote the development of Global Public Goods (GPGs) for health, which can provide enduring benefits for all countries and all people. This approach includes such actions as medical research and development focused on diseases that most affect the poor. In addition, trade in goods and services and multilateral trade agreements have an increasing influence on the health of the poor. Of particular significance are those agreements dealing with trade related aspects of intellectual property rights (TRIPS), the General Agreement on Trade in Services (GATS), and trade in hazardous substances.*

1. Introduction

The health problems of the poor do not stop at national borders. In a globalised world, people and information as well as goods and services travel across borders with increasing speed and ease. Globalisation thus presents new risks to health, as is indicated by the rapid spread of HIV/AIDS or the threat of bioterrorism. Yet it also provides new opportunities to prevent, treat or contain disease. National governments, working at the regional and global levels, must devise new ways of working together to address common threats to health.

At the national level, coherent PRSs focus on health outcomes and other MDGs and include the role of policies and programmes in all policy areas relevant to the health of the poor and the performance of health systems (see Chapter 4). These include economic and fiscal policies, which influence the real incomes of poor people and the price of goods and services affecting health, as well as the private and public revenues available for health expenditure. In addition, rules and policies governing international trade in goods and services play a major role in determining the availability and affordability of essential health inputs – especially pharmaceutical products – for poor people and countries.

Chapter 5 focuses on two key aspects of international co-operation that complement and reinforce the efforts of national governments to improve the health of the poor. First, it considers global public goods (GPGs) for the benefit of public health everywhere, particularly in low-income countries. Second, it deals with the links between international trade agreements and the health of poor people, particularly the agreements dealing with trade-related intellectual property rights, trade in health services, and trade in hazardous substances. Another important aspect concerns the health implications of migration.

Development agencies have important roles to play in fostering international collective action to improve the health of the poor. They can help to strengthen capacity in low-income countries to contribute to the development of GPGs for health. They can encourage support for international initiatives that bring together developed and developing countries along with representatives of the private sector and civil society – including "public-private partnerships" – to create new incentives and boost commitment to reducing the burden of disease in partner countries. They can foster policy dialogue and provide technical assistance to developing country officials, especially in the health and trade sectors, in order to promote national policy coherence. Finally, they can be advocates within their own governments on global policy coherence issues – ranging from health research to trade and migration policy – relevant to poverty and health.

2. Global Public Goods for health

The importance of GPGs has been increasingly recognised in international development circles. The concept is used in various ways – from the definition of public goods in economic theory as non-rival and non-excludable to "goods with benefits that extend to all countries, people, and generations".[1] The term "global public goods" is used here as in evolving international practice to denote products, services and conditions that are under-supplied by the market, are of broad international concern, and require international public action.

GPGs for health can be provided only by countries working together, often in partnership with the private sector. The challenge facing development agencies is how to call government-wide attention to the benefit that GPGs for health can bring to all people and countries. The following sub-sections describe two examples of global public goods for health, and identify what is required to strengthen the incentives for providing them: i) research and development for more effective health systems, and ii) effective public-health surveillance to detect and control the cross-border spread of communicable diseases. There are other GPGs for health, which are not discussed in any detail here. These include health commodity security,[3] global action to promote information and communication technology and management (ICT/ICM) and other forms of knowledge about how best to organise and finance health services to improve health outcomes among the poor. (This reference document is a case in point.)

2.1. Research and development

The generation and dissemination of knowledge in the health system is central to disease prevention and treatment. Poor countries benefit least from research and development (R&D) of new drugs, vaccines and diagnostics. They are also least able to finance public investment into R&D, and their markets lack the purchasing power to motivate private-sector research against the diseases that are prevalent locally in these countries.

It is estimated that less than 10% of global spending on health research is devoted to diseases or conditions that account for 90% of the global disease burden.[4] In defining priorities for bridging this "10:90 gap", incentives have to be matched with particular diseases. In this regard, a useful distinction was made by the CMH between three categories of diseases:[5]

- **Diseases common in both rich and poor countries** such as diabetes, hepatitis B and measles, for which incentives for private R&D already exist. The question is rather how to make the prices for newly invented drugs and vaccines to treat these diseases affordable to poor people in low-income countries. One way is voluntary or negotiated systems of differential pricing for drugs, in which poor countries pay lower prices and rich countries higher ones for expensive drugs under patent protection. Development agencies might consider ways of promoting this solution, which was endorsed by the CMH, within their own governments and in international forums. Where differential pricing mechanisms do not work, and prices for patented drugs remain beyond the reach of poor countries, some remedies may be possible through trade arrangements, as discussed in Section 3.

- **Diseases common in both rich and poor countries but with the largest affected populations in the low-income countries**, such as HIV/AIDS. For these diseases, R&D incentives exist but the investment volume is disproportionate to the burden of disease in low-income countries. In this situation, a combination of "push" (support to research per se) and "pull" (support to research by increasing demand for the products to be developed from research) incentives may be necessary. More public investment in global R&D in diseases that primarily affect poor people – channelled through international coalitions that can identify priorities and promising initiatives – could push the private sector and research communities to spend more on these diseases. In some cases, commitments to purchase new drugs and vaccines targeted on neglected diseases might pull the R&D process faster along.

● **Diseases specific to poor countries in tropical climates**, such as malaria, Chagas disease, sleeping sickness and onchocercosis (river blindness). For these diseases, even stronger efforts may be necessary to induce new R&D. Here increased public funding of basic biomedical research is necessary as well as the "push" and "pull" measures described above. One promising approach that merits further examination would be to extend programmes already in place in OECD countries for their own "orphan diseases" to cover diseases of developing countries as well. Orphan-drug incentive programmes can include research grants, tax credits, or extensions of patent protection.[6]

Aligning the incentives to stimulate R&D investment on diseases that primarily affect the poor in low-income countries requires international co-operation and close collaboration between public and private sectors. Currently, there is a wealth of initiatives under way to encourage vitally necessary but under-provided medical R&D, but the share of research going to the health problems of poorer countries remains well below what is needed.[7]

Such initiatives are often based in multilateral institutions (WHO, UNAIDS, UNDP or the World Bank), but they increasingly involve partnerships between international agencies, pharmaceutical companies, private non-profit organisations, bilateral aid agencies, research institutions and private foundations. When appropriately organised and motivated, such public-private partnerships (PPPs) constitute a key strategy in tackling neglected health issues in developing countries.

The CMH also proposed that funding be provided for a potential Global Health Research Fund (GHRF) – in effect, an international version of National Institutes of Health or Medical Research Councils within OECD countries. Appropriate governance of the GHRF would then become an important issue.

2.2. Cross-border spread of communicable diseases

Increased travel, migration, and trade in food and animals across borders make the world more vulnerable to the cross-border spread of communicable diseases. In addition to medical R&D, cross-border surveillance, prevention and control constitutes a key GPG for health. Three types of international collective action can help prevent cross-border transmission of disease: disease surveillance, the containment of anti-microbial resistance (AMR), and disease eradication programmes. The effectiveness of all three activities depends largely on national and regional capacity. Low capacity or weak performance in one country is a threat to all and so production of the GPG in this instance calls for efforts to strengthen the weakest links in the control chain for communicable diseases.

Global and national disease surveillance

The first step in controlling the transmission of disease across international borders is to detect it. Countries have been co-operating in efforts to monitor and track the spread of communicable disease for more than a century. The WHO's global outbreak alert and verification process, epidemic preparedness plans and stockpiles of essential medicines have reduced the call on trade embargoes or travel restrictions to control cross-border disease transmission. Nonetheless, the current system is still fragmented and suffers from chronic under-funding. Low-income countries are the weakest link in the global chain of surveillance: they lack sufficient laboratories and technicians, communications infrastructure, and disease reporting systems; linkages between monitoring and response systems are also inadequate.

Efforts to address the problems in low-income countries have been under way for many years, assisted by WHO and development agency support. They require further attention. But better-trained health professionals cannot compensate for a global system that is inadequate to deal with the challenges presented by the emergence of new pathogens, the re-emergence of old ones, and the development of drug-resistant strains of microbes.

In 1995 the WHO started the process of revising the International Health Regulations (IHR), currently the only international health treaty, expanding the scope of notifications required of WHO member States beyond just plague, cholera, and yellow fever, to cover *"public health emergencies of international concern"*. Low-income countries require support to participate fully in the IHR negotiations and, once the revised IHR is adopted, to implement changes required in their surveillance systems.

Global strategies for containing anti-microbial resistance

The ability of micro-organisms to develop resistance to antibiotics is a natural biological occurrence, but it has been exacerbated by the improper use of antibiotics. Resistance to antiretroviral therapy for HIV/AIDS is an issue of rapidly growing concern. In several countries, tuberculosis strains have become resistant to at least two of the most effective drugs used against the disease. Elsewhere, commonly used anti-malarial drugs have become virtually useless because the malaria parasite has acquired resistance to them – and when treatment fails, patients remain infective for longer periods of time, increasing the opportunity for the resistant strain to spread. Drugs needed to treat multi drug-resistant TB are nearly 100 times more expensive than drugs used to treat non-resistant strains.

Action taken in any one country may benefit all. Overuse of antibiotics is a global concern, while misuse and underuse are more important problems in many developing countries. International collective action is important for setting norms and standards to facilitate responsible national policies. In 2001, the WHO launched a global strategy to contain the spread of drug resistance, involving over 50 recommendations for patients, health providers, hospital managers, health ministers and agricultural-sector policy makers and managers (antibiotics used for disease control and growth promotion in animals contributes to drug resistance in humans).

Because most of the responsibility for implementing the recommendations lies with national governments, it is in the interest of DAC members to provide assistance to low-income countries which lack the resources to take the necessary action. Strengthening their capacity for pharmaceutical regulation, including the surveillance of the use of anti-microbial drugs and containment of drug resistance, is an example of a global public health good that merits broad development agency support.

Disease eradication and elimination programmes

Eradication is often cited as an example of a "pure" global public good: once eradication has been achieved, all countries gain and they do not have to compete for their share of the benefits. There are also clear and lasting benefits to eradication: since the final eradication of smallpox in 1979, an estimated 30 million lives and USD 275 million in annual direct costs have been saved.

Eradication of polio is now 99% complete, largely thanks to national mass immunisation campaigns, supported by a global coalition of international organisations and bilateral development agencies and civil society organisations. Once polio has been eradicated, savings on vaccination costs worldwide will amount to over USD 1 billion a year. The benefits of disease-control efforts are biggest for countries which have already reduced prevalence rates of diseases within their borders to relatively low figures. Yet, only through global elimination will the costs incurred by that disease disappear. For example, the United States stands to save around USD 250 million a year – the amount it now spends on polio immunisation every year to prevent the re-importation of a disease it has already eradicated.

A number of other diseases are amenable to eradication or elimination. Available and effective prevention or treatment is a precondition, as are sufficient means and motivation to extend vaccines or treatment to all. In addition to polio, global efforts are focused on eliminating (or reducing the number of cases to less than 1 in 10 000 in the total population) filariasis, leprosy, guinea-worm disease, tetanus, Chagas disease, and measles. Development co-operation has helped to supplement these disease control initiatives in low-income countries. The resources that have been made available are nonetheless still small relative to the amounts required. More effort is necessary, both nationally and internationally, as these initiatives get closer to achieving their goals.

2.3. GPGs for Health – recommendations for development agencies

Development agencies have a central role to play in correcting the "incentive gap" for the production of global public goods for health. Recent developments suggest that appeals for financing and developing GPGs help increase support for aid for health and for aid overall. Since the benefits derived from GPGs for health accrue to rich countries as well as poor, *funding for GPGs should come, to the extent feasible, from sources other than ODA* (*e.g.* national health sector or research budgets in OECD countries, as well as in part from increased international aid budgets). This diversity of sources could provide enlarged funding and technical support to help tackle critical global health problems. Increased aid effectiveness requires, in part, assisting the achievement of enhanced GPGs for health.

Development co-operation agencies can help to close the gap between current R&D investment and the health problems of the poor by *supporting under-funded activities in low-income countries that are important to ensure global health benefits*. This would strengthen the capacity of developing countries to participate as partners in the production of GPGs for health, involving, for example:

- **Assisting partner countries to develop the institutions necessary for testing new health technologies** and using them effectively.

- **Fostering collaboration between research institutions** in developed and developing countries for R&D on GPGs, with a focus on neglected diseases, and encouraging financial support for regional research and training centres.

- **Promoting policy dialogue** among developed and developing countries to help create an enabling environment for the provision of GPGs.

- **Encouraging medical research councils in developing countries to focus more on the diseases of the poor** and support institutions that co-ordinate such research on a global scale.

- **Supporting low-income countries' participation in the IHR revision** process to ensure that their needs and priorities are reflected and helping with the implementation of any required changes in their surveillance systems.

- **Strengthening national disease surveillance systems**, to contain AMR and implement disease eradication and elimination programmes.

Development agencies can also provide critical financial support to international initiatives seeking to produce new vaccines, drugs and knowledge focused on the health problems of the poor. According to the CMH, USD 3 billion is required by 2007 and USD 4 billion by 2015 for the development of new vaccines and drugs. It is important that this funding be consistent. It can come through direct funding and through the range of "push" and "pull" incentives, including through "orphan drug" programmes discussed above. They can also urge other relevant government agencies, in a push for policy coherence, to give higher priority in health research to diseases of importance to developing countries.

Consideration should also be given to pilot projects to pre-commit funds to buy products of new research. These projects should include expert purchasers, negotiating with pharmaceutical companies to obtain the lowest viable commercial price.

3. Health, trade and development

Trade in goods and services has an increasingly important impact on the health of the poor. Thus, the global, regional and bilateral agreements that govern international trade are relevant to this document, and warrant a brief overview so that development agencies can engage in discussions with government trade departments about policy coherence for global health. The scope of trade and health issues is large;[8] this section focuses on: i) intellectual property rights and access to essential pharmaceutical products; ii) trade in services and its implications for access to health services by the poor; and (ii) trade in hazardous commodities.

3.1. Intellectual property rights and access to essential medicines

- **The importance of ensuring affordable access for poor countries and people to essential drugs and vaccines** is emphasised in the UN Millennium Declaration and reflected in the MDGs.[9] Such access depends on several critical elements, including effective pro-poor health systems, rational selection and use, affordable prices, sustainable financing and reliable supply and delivery systems. Several of these factors are discussed above, and this section focuses on the issue of price in the context of trade agreements. Lowering the price of essential medicines is vital to pro-poor health in developing countries. Their share of spending on pharmaceuticals in total health expenditures is high (25 to 65%), yet the health budgets of developing countries are generally too small to finance programmes to ensure access for poor people to essential medicines.

The World Trade Organization (WTO) Agreement on *Trade-Related Aspects of Intellectual Property Rights (TRIPS)* provides at least 20 years of patent protection for all inventions of products and processes in all WTO member countries, although transition periods are granted for developing countries and, in particular, for the least developed countries. The patent confers on its owner the exclusive right to make, use, offer for sale, sell, or import the patented products. This monopoly usually involves much higher prices during the period of patent protection, before generic competition is allowed. For the pharmaceutical industry, patent protection is vital in the recovery of R&D costs and as an incentive for the development of new medicines.

Yet the importance of patent protection, relative to other constraints, including inadequate demand and institutional issues in low-income countries, should not be exaggerated. Most of the essential drugs listed by the WHO are already in the public domain, because they have either never been patented or their patents have expired. Although patent protection for pharmaceutical products is available in most developing countries, companies have not patented their products in all of them, especially in the least developed countries and other countries with small markets or limited technological capacity. They will have to import such products either from countries where patent protection applies or, if possible, from countries where the products are not patented. *Parallel importation* is not covered by the TRIPS Agreement. This concept refers to importing, at a lower price, patented or trademarked products from countries where it is marketed by the rights holder.

● **The TRIPS Agreement states as a principle the right to adopt measures necessary to protect public health and nutrition** and to promote the public interest in sectors of vital importance to their socio-economic and technological development, provided that such measures are consistent with the provisions of the Agreement. It also provides limited exceptions to the exclusive rights conferred by a patent, *e.g.* for the protection of human life or health. This may include *compulsory licensing*, whereby a government can authorise production of a patented product or use a patented process without the consent of the patent owner in the case of a national emergency.

The WTO Ministerial Conference in Qatar in November 2001 adopted the *Doha Declaration on the TRIPS Agreement and Public Health*, which made a number of important clarifications. It affirmed that each WTO member has the right to grant compulsory licences and the freedom to determine the grounds upon which such licences are granted. Further, each member has the right to use patents in the case of national emergencies without the authorisation of the rights holder, and to determine what constitutes a national emergency or other circumstances of extreme urgency. It was understood that these may include public health crises relating to *e.g.* HIV/AIDS, tuberculosis, malaria and other epidemics.

TRIPS compulsory licensing rules require that products made under such licences be "authorised predominantly for the supply of the domestic market of the member authorising such use" (Article 31.f). The Doha Declaration recognised that WTO members with insufficient or no manufacturing capacities in the pharmaceutical sector could face difficulties in making effective use of compulsory licensing under the TRIPS Agreement, and instructed the Council for TRIPS to find an expeditious solution to this problem.[10] The WTO has also extended the transition period for the least developed countries until 2016 for the obligation to grant patents in the pharmaceutical sector.

● **Member agencies should encourage their governments to monitor the implementation of the Doha Declaration on TRIPS and Public Health,** including the outcome of efforts by the WTO Council to find a solution to the problems of certain countries to make effective use of compulsory licensing. It is important to assess the capability of developing countries, in particular low-income countries, to use the TRIPS Agreement for improving their access, at affordable prices, to pro-poor health priority medicines under patent protection.

3.2. International trade and migration – health implications

International trade in health services is rising, driven by a multitude of factors. Advances in communications technology make it possible to deliver telemedicine across borders while giving rise to new forms of trade in health services, such as providing diagnoses and treatment advice to clinics in low-income countries. Faster and less costly travel makes it easier to obtain care in other countries, and developing countries are marketing special packages to attract medical "tourists". Health care reforms in some countries have created opportunities for private suppliers – domestic and foreign-owned – to provide services. And increasing numbers of health professionals are migrating, temporarily or permanently, from lower to higher-income countries in search of higher wages and better working conditions.

The WTO *General Agreement on Trade in Services (GATS)* provides WTO members with a range of policy options to allow them to liberalise services trade on a gradual basis, in line with their development objectives. GATS negotiations under way in the WTO aim to achieve progressively higher degrees of liberalisation of trade in services. The negotiations do not exclude *a priori* any service sector, although each WTO member is free to choose which sectors it will liberalise and the extent of liberalisation it will undertake there. In determining whether or to what extent they wish to liberalise trade in health services, WTO members need to consider the potential benefits and risks to poor people's access to health services.

Increased foreign investment in private health facilities may improve the quality of care in recipient countries, especially in the tertiary sector (*i.e.* university or highly specialised hospital services). But if this investment is on a large scale and supports hospitals and services that offer more attractive wages and working conditions, it may exacerbate medical and nursing staff shortages in the rural and public facilities on which poor people rely. The lack of empirical evidence on the impact of privatisation (which GATS does not cover) on access to health services by the poor in low-income countries suggests that more research and monitoring is called for. Lessons from other sectors on the sequencing of reform suggest that the achievement of pro-poor health goals requires that countries put effective regulatory frameworks in place *before* privatisation and opening the market to foreign investors.

There is a general lack of adequately trained staff in low-income countries. It is essential that the capacity of professional medical staff in these countries should be enhanced through improved working conditions, in particular the rehabilitation of facilities and equipment, reforms in the management of human resources, support schemes and reintegration of private-sector practitioners into public-sector systems. North-South institutional partnerships can contribute here, through documentation and training programmes, among other means.

Health professionals often emigrate to benefit from better salaries and working conditions. Such emigration may be temporary or permanent, which raises different issues for both sending and receiving countries. Yet their professional education has usually been highly subsidised to enhance the supply of qualified staff in their own health systems. In only a few countries (the Philippines is one) could it be reasonably argued that remittances substantially offset the cost of reducing the domestic supply of health professionals.

Some OECD countries facing their own shortages of professional staff have encouraged migration, with active recruitment of people from/in developing countries with appropriate professional and language skills. Unless explicitly considered and mitigated, this practice will have repercussions on the capacity problems of health systems in the source countries exacerbating their shortages of professional staff. Some OECD countries are taking steps to address these issues, particularly that of active recruitment, and to enhance policy coherence for pro-poor health. It has also been suggested that WHO develop an ethical chart on the international recruitment of health professionals, including support for improved employment conditions in low-income source countries.

As international trade in health services grows and diversifies, and as agreements concerning services trade expand to cover health care, developing countries require capacity and assistance on how to assess the benefits and risks, and the implications for the regulation of health systems. Development agencies may consider how to support the needs of low-income countries for specialised technical assistance on trade in health services and encourage dialogue between health and trade ministries to ensure national policy coherence. Agencies might also search for opportunities to support credible research on the effects of trade liberalisation on access to health services by the poor, to expand the body of knowledge on this issue.

3.3. Trade in hazardous commodities

International trade in goods, products and commodities may involve public health concerns. The WTO allows its members to make exceptions to the rules of free trade in order to protect human life or health and to protect the environment, even if manufacturers assert that the risk can be contained.[11] There are several international treaties that address trade in hazardous goods, reflecting the international community's common concern and responsibility for tackling transboundary or global environmental problems that affect human health.[12]

A Framework Convention on Tobacco Control (FCTC) is currently being proposed.[13] Among its trade-related features are those designed to: combat illegal trade and smuggling; phase out duty-free sales and increase and harmonise taxes internationally; exempt tobacco products from reduced tariff agreements; and address various packaging, labelling and advertising issues.

Development agencies concerned to promote the health of the poor in developing countries through measures to reduce exposure to hazardous goods and commodities, including tobacco, should consult with colleagues in environment and trade departments. Such discussions should seek coherence in OECD country policies on aid, trade, environment and health.

Notes

1. The definition quoted in Kaul, P., P. Conceiçao, K. Le Goulven and R. Mendoza (eds.) (undated), *Providing Global Public Goods, Managing Globalization*, p.26. Accessible at *www.undp.org/ globalpublicgoods/globalization/toc.html* .

2. *"Non-excludability"* means that it is either impossible or prohibitively costly to exclude those who do not pay for consuming a good or service; *"Non-rivalry"* means that one person's consumption of a public good has no effect on the amount available to others. The corresponding concept of a *"public bad"* refers to goods or services that have a negative utility, which the community would benefit from preventing or reducing.

3. That is the supply of condoms and other contraceptives required to achieve internationally agreed goals on reproductive health.

4. The Global Forum for Health Research (2002), *The 10/90 Report on Health Research 2001-2002.* Geneva. Accessible at *www.globalforumhealth.org*

5. WHO (2001), *Macroeconomics and Health: Investing in Health for Economic Development, Report of the Commission on Macroeconomics and Health,* WHO, Geneva.

6. "Orphan diseases" are those with such low incidence in developed countries that market incentives to induce R&D are lacking.

7. For a review of some of these initiatives, see *The Global Forum for Health Research (2002), op. cit.,* Chapter 8, "Some networks in the priority research areas".

8. See the report, WHO/WTO (2002), *WTO Agreements and Public Health: A Joint Report by the WHO and WTO Secretariats.* Accessible at *www.who.int/media/homepage/who_wto_e.pdf*

9. MDG Goal 8: "Develop a global partnership for development"; Target 17: "In co-operation with pharmaceutical companies, provide access to affordable, essential drugs in developing countries".

10. As of February 2003, no solution had been agreed by the TRIPS Council.

11. A recent dispute taken to the WTO involving asbestos – a well-established carcinogen – affirmed that countries could ban trade in goods hazardous to health. An account of this case is provided in WHO/WTO (2002), *op. cit.*

12. These include the Basel Convention on the Transboundary Movement of Hazardous Wastes, the Rotterdam Convention on Prior Informed Consent (PIC) for dangerous chemicals and the Stockholm Convention on Persistent Organic Pollutants (POPs).

13. See Chapter 2, Box 2. The FCTC is being negotiated and is expected to be ready to be submitted for signature by participating governments in 2003.

ISBN 92-64-10018-0
DAC Guidelines and Reference Documents
Poverty and Health
© OECD, WHO 2003

Bibliography

Asian Development Bank (2001),
Attacking the Double Burden of Malnutrition in Asia and the Pacific. Asian Development Bank, Manila. Accessible at *www.adb.org/documents/books/nutrition/malnutrition/default.asp*

Bennett, S. and L. Gilson (2001),
Health Financing: Designing and Implementing Pro-poor Schemes, DFID Health Systems Resource Centre, London, Accessible at *www.healthsystemsrc.org*

CIDA (Canadian International Development Agency) (2001),
CIDA's Draft Action Plan on Health and Nutrition, CIDA, May 2001.

Commission of the European Communities (2002),
Health and Poverty Reduction in Developing Countries, Communication from the Commission to the Council and the European Parliament, Brussels, COM(2002)129 Final. Accessible at *www.europa.eu.int/eur-lex/en/com/cnc/2002/com2002_0129en01.pdf*

Diamond, I., Z. Matthews and R. Stephenson (2001),
Assessing the Health of the Poor: Towards a Pro-poor Measurement Strategy, DFID Health Systems Resource Centre, London. Accessible at *www.healthsystemsrc.org*

DFID (2000),
Better Health for Poor People, Issues paper, DFID, London. Accessible at *www.dfid.gov.uk/pubs/files/tsp_health.pdf*

GTZ (Deutsche Gesellschaft für Technische Zusammenarbeit) (2002),
Die Dinge beim Namen nennen – Gewalt gegen Frauen im Alltag, (Telling it Like it Is – Violence Against Women in Everyday Life). Accessible at *www.gtz.de*

IFPRI (International Food Policy Research Institute) (2000),
"Overcoming Child Malnutrition in Developing Countries", *Food, Agriculture and the Environment Discussion Paper No. 30,* IFPRI, Washington.

Inter-Agency Group on Sector-Wide Approaches for Health Development (2001),
Orientation and Training Seminars for Agency Staff: Sector-Wide Approaches for Health in a Changing Environment: Seminar Handbook, IHSD Ltd., London.

International Monetary Fund/World Bank (2001),
Poverty Reduction Strategy Papers – Progress in Implementation, DC2001-0010, IMF/World Bank, Washington.

JICA (Japanese International Co-operation Agency) (2001),
Lusaka District Primary Health Care Project in Zambia, Project Evaluation Report, JICA.

OECD (2000),
Shaping the Urban Environment in the 21st Century: From Understanding to Action, DAC/OECD, Paris.

OECD (2000),
Resource Book for Urban Development and Co-operation 2000, OECD, Paris.

OECD (2002),
"Health, Education and Poverty Reduction", *OECD Development Centre, Policy Brief No. 19,* OECD, Paris.

SIDA (Swedish International Development Agency) (2001),
Health and Environment, SIDA, Stockholm.

SIDA (2002),
Health is Wealth, draft, SIDA, Stockholm.

UNDP (United Nations Development Program) (2000),
  Attacking Poverty While Improving the Environment: Towards Win-Win Policy Options, Poverty and Environment Initiative, UNDP/EC.

USAID (United States Agency for International Development) (n.d.),
  Serving the Poor: The USAID Global Health Experience in Poverty Reduction, internal document, USAID, Washington.

World Bank (2001),
  Making Sustainable Commitments: An Environment Strategy for the World Bank, World Bank, Washington.

World Bank (2002),
  World Development Indicators 2002, World Bank, Washington.

World Bank (2002),
  Millennium Development Goals, World Bank, Washington.

WHO, (World Health Organization) (1997),
  The World Health Report 1997: Conquering Suffering, Enriching Humanity, WHO, Geneva.

WHO (1999),
  The World Health Report 1999: Making a Difference, WHO, Geneva.

WHO (2000),
  Health: A Precious Asset, Accelerating Follow-up to the World Summit for Social Development, Proposals by WHO, WHO, Geneva (WHO/HSD/HID/00.1).

WHO (2000),
  Sector-Wide Approaches for Health Development: A Review of Experience, Strategies for Co-operation and Partnership, Global Programme on Evidence for Health Policy, WHO, Geneva.

WHO (2001),
  Macroeconomics and Health: Investing in Health for Economic Development, Report of the Commission on Macroeconomics and Health, WHO, Geneva.

WHO (2001),
  Review of Implementation and Effectiveness of Existing Policy Instruments on Transport, Environment and Health, and of their Potential for Health Gain, WHO, Geneva.

DAC GUIDELINES AND REFERENCE DOCUMENTS: POVERTY AND HEALTH – ISBN 92-64-10018-0 – © OECD, WHO 2003